HOPE BEYOND HIGH-RISK MULTIPLE MYELOMA

A Personal Diary

Denny C. Davis

Copyright © 2020 by Denny C. Davis
All rights reserved.

Independently published in the United States of America
Kindle-Amazon Direct Printing

Author contact
DennyCDavis73@gmail.com
http://VerityDesignLearning.com

Dedication

This book is dedicated to the many medical professionals who day after day invest themselves selflessly in the lives of cancer patients. Their skillful care, compassion, and encouragement give patients a measure of hope. The book is also dedicated to the Great Physician who gives sure hope for traveling through daily trials and for all of eternity.

Acknowledgements

The author would like to thank the many friends and family members who have encouraged and prayed for me through my cancer journey and through the preparation of this book. Special thanks go to my wife Irma who is always my greatest encourager; her timely nudges and frank feedback have kept me moving to goal completion. Indirectly, Tom Brokaw encouraged me through his book describing his lucky life interrupted by multiple myeloma. Special thanks to Megan Orme who read my book with a medical practitioner's eye and helped me see its value to medical professionals.

I especially thank Almighty God who enabled me to travel the multiple myeloma journey amazingly well and who gives me hope for the future. Words of strength and assurance from His holy Scriptures provided an anchor that held me secure through stormy times. God's promise that He works through trials to produce good in His people is so reassuring.

Table of Contents

PROLOGUE 1
INTRODUCTION 3
SURPRISE DIAGNOSIS 6
CRANIAL SURGERY 13
PREPARATION FOR CHEMO 18
CHEMOTHERAPY PHASE 1 22
CANCER REMISSION 35
TRANSPLANT DECISION 41
HARVESTING STEM CELLS 45
STEM CELL TRANSPLANT 52
TRANSPLANT VALLEY 64
OUTPATIENT RECOVERY 80
PARTIAL REMISSION 95
A SURE HOPE 108

Prologue
Opening Perspective

The word "cancer" sends chills up the spine. How does one prepare to fight this mortal enemy . . be it real or imagined?

This is a personal account of a hope-filled encounter with multiple myeloma. I begin with a brief description of my life as a retired university professor, unexpectedly breached by news that I had multiple myeloma. I share diary entries to detail my cancer diagnosis, treatment experiences, and thoughts. I conclude with insights about how God's personal care gives one hope that permeates and transcends the multiple myeloma journey.

A backdrop to this story is found in the Bible (James 1:2-4, NKJV):

> *"Count it all joy when you fall into various trials, knowing that the testing of your faith produces patience. But let patience have its perfect work, that you may be perfect and complete, lacking nothing."*

If this is true, tough life experiences have potential to refine and complete one's life, helping us to finish strong! As a Christian, I found from this statement assurance that helped me interpret and successfully navigate my cancer experiences.

My desire is to help others (cancer patients, people close to a patient, and medical professionals working with cancer patients) to successfully walk the tortuous cancer journey. Perhaps you can see from my experiences how cancer can affect the patient's life, emotions, relationships, and views of the future. But also realize that my encounter with multiple myeloma will not be what everyone else experiences, and my interpretations of medical conditions could be flawed.

However, there is hope. Be encouraged! When facing trials from multiple myeloma or other life disrupting events, you can live your life and help others live their lives with tangible, lasting hope.

Introduction
Introducing the Author

When retiring in May 2012 from a 36-year career in engineering education at Washington State University (WSU), I entered a life stage that I knew would end. I didn't think much about when or how it might end, but I knew that death would come and it might be from failing health. Perhaps my lack of concern was because I had peace with the Creator and Sustainer of all things. I knew that God watches over me and will usher me into eternity with Him when I die.

In my university years, I had been a worker, so I probably needed retirement goals. But I entered retirement without a bucket list or set of aspirations to reach new heights of excellence. I felt that God would lead me to purposeful activities that probably involved family nearby. I had not considered that my final years might be crafted by my Creator to prepare me for eternity. Neither did I know that multiple myeloma had a role in the completion process.

This book presents my multiple myeloma journey in the context of other dimensions of my life: interactions with family, professional contributions in engineering education, and motivations to develop and make productive the place where I lived with my wife.

My story begins in early 2018, happily married to my wife Irma for nearly 46 years. We had moved to Mascoutah, Illinois in 2011 to be near our only offspring Nancy, her husband Josh, and their seven (now nine) children.

We lived two doors away from Josh, Nancy, and the kids. They are a musical family. Parents and children old enough are competent in voice as well as piano and one or more additional instruments. Nancy home educates the children. Josh operates a home improvement business as his principal source of income. Being near our family gave us opportunities for sharing special events in life and for helping one another.

Irma and I lived in a 4,500 square foot ranch style house that suffered many remodels by previous owners, and we did our share to fix it up. Our 1-acre lot had a large in-ground swimming pool, an oak tree shaded yard, and struggling garden areas sporting fruit trees, berries, and other crops. We fought a battle with squirrels, raccoons, and other small critters who stole our produce. In fact, I trapped eight raccoons in our yard during a 2-week period in 2017. I had been stopped by police officers more than once for using electric fence and an air rifle to keep critters out of my garden.

I carried remnants of my university teaching, curriculum development, and educational research into retirement. For decades I had collaborated with educators across the nation to develop teaching materials and assessments to improve student learning of engineering design and professional skills. Upon retirement, I created workbooks and card decks to guide student discussions, reflections, and assessments that grew their skills in teamwork, professional responsibility, design, and professional behaviors. I formed a company, Verity Design Learning, which published and marketed my materials.

After moving to Illinois, I began coaching in the FIRST® (For Inspiration and Recognition of Science and Technology) program because my oldest grandson was involved and I saw how I could use my engineering education experience to help kids learn. Immediately I co-coached a FIRST Lego League (FLL) team for middle school students. When my grandson aged out of FLL, I "graduated" to coaching FIRST Tech Challenge (FTC) for high school students.

Since 2015, our home school FTC team has met in our home, using half of our garage for their shop and our playroom for meeting space. With four skilled coaches and motivated kids, the Robo Raiders FTC 7129 have done exceptionally well—advancing to state, super regional, and world competition levels multiple years.

My faith has been an important part of my life leading up to my multiple myeloma story. Since 1969 when God changed my life from aimlessness to one of purpose and hope, I have sought to honor and obey Him. For nearly 50 years I found Jesus Christ's promise trustworthy (John 10:10b, NKJV):

> "I have come that they may have life, and that they may have it more abundantly".

I had indeed experienced a life that was full of meaning and good things. I also believed the biblical promise (Romans 8:28):

> "And we know that all things work together for good to those who love God, to those who are the called according to His purpose".

I had received many good things in life; when hard times came, they eventually worked to good ends. I assumed that my retirement years would similarly see God's faithful guidance and support through unknown conditions to reach good ends.

This sets the stage for my story. I had enjoyed a full and productive life. Multiple myeloma invaded my life in early 2018 amid a busy and productive retirement. My diary documents how multiple myeloma took front stage in my life while other responsibilities continued. I end with my attempt to make sense of this drama and highlight the hope that strengthens and refines us for a wonderful future after cancer deals its final blow.

Surprise Diagnosis
What is Multiple Myeloma?

My cancer diagnosis was a huge surprise to me. It began in an annual checkup with my family doctor. I did not expect anything out of the ordinary to result from this visit, but this was just the first step in a long, uncertain journey.

Monday, February 12, 2018

First thing Monday morning I met with Dr. Pritchett, to review blood test results and discuss my general health. All appeared to be very good. Near the end of my appointment, I pointed out a sizable lump on the back of my head that I had noticed over the past few weeks. When Dr. Pritchett felt the lump, he told me it felt strange and I should have it scanned. He arranged an appointment for a CT scan.

Wednesday, February 14, 2018

On Wednesday, Valentine's Day, I drove to St. Elizabeth's Hospital, 13 miles away, for a 9:45 am scan. Because I considered this routine, I drove myself and expected to be home in short order. A technician completed one scan, showed it to a second person, and took another scan from a slightly different angle. Then I was escorted to the waiting area.

A few minutes later, the technician brought a wheel chair and instructed me to hop in. She said the scan showed a mass that had eroded a hole in my skull and was pressing on my brain. They were admitting me to the emergency room (ER) while they arranged for an ambulance to transport me to St Louis where neurologists could further study the mass and perform surgery if necessary. The urgency of my condition caught me totally off guard because I had no symptoms that might be expected when an object presses on the brain. I had absolutely no fear as I followed their instructions and considered what to do.

During ER check-in, I called Irma and told her what was happening. I asked her to get help from Nancy so they could come see what was happening and get our car.

Some of our Robo Raiders robotics team was to meet at our house that afternoon, so I contacted the other coaches/mentors and told them of my situation. Irma left the door unlocked so they could get in the house for their 3 to 6 pm meeting.

Irma and Nancy quickly came to the hospital to check on me and get our car. After an hour in ER, a neurosurgery room became available at St Louis University Hospital (SLUH) and I was transported there by ambulance. Even though I faced a serious medical condition, my confidence in God gave me peace that surpassed my understanding and kept me from worrying.

Irma and Nancy went home, taking our car as well. Nancy then drove the two of them to SLUH where they found me in ER. Medical personnel repeatedly asked me about pain, dizziness, and limited movement in my limbs– symptoms usually resulting from brain trauma that they expected. I had none of these symptoms. In fact, I felt normal and had no pathological symptoms from the large tumor. Finally, I was moved to a room in the neurosurgery floor.

That afternoon medical staff scanned my head, lungs, and pelvis and took multiple blood samples. As test results became available, I heard things I did not understand, but I thought I heard the word "cancer" among them. Biopsies and additional tests would be used to make a more certain diagnosis.

As the day progressed, I was told that I might have multiple myeloma in the large mass in my skull and in my right hip where a small lesion was identified. Multiple myeloma was described as cancer of the blood plasma, originating in bone marrow, and very mobile. It often goes to sites in bones and creates lesions there, weakening bones and making them susceptible to fractures. It also can be very painful in sites where it is present.

An MRI of my brain resulted in a report (excerpt shown), which gave the size of the tumor and named multiple myeloma as a likely diagnosis. When the doctor told me what was found, I was amazed at the size of the mass and its likelihood of being cancerous. Although I wondered what this might mean for me and my family, I was not afraid. I wondered where God would take us and how He might use this in our lives.

> 2/14/2018 MRI BRAIN: ... mass centered on the occipital bone with midline measuring 3.8 x 7.5 x 9.1 cm which expands and erodes occipital and parietal bones and places mass effect on the underlying occipital lobes and cerebellum without evidence of intraparenchymal invasion or adjacent edema. Differential considerations include such processes as ... multiple myeloma.

That afternoon we informed Pastor Steve from our church so he was aware of our situation. That evening Irma emailed her older sister to inform her of my condition.

Thursday, February 15, 2018

Irma and Nancy stayed home, waiting to see if I would be discharged or taken into emergency surgery. Medical teams from neurology, neurosurgery, oncology, and hematology called for tests to diagnose my cancer with certainty, locate other lesions, and assess the extent of its invasion into other parts of my body. I had several x-ray, CT, and MRI scans that afternoon and into the night.

Evidence was mounting that I had multiple myeloma. A test called a serum free light chain test was used to measure small amounts of kappa and lambda light chain proteins in the blood. If myeloma cells made either free kappa or lambda light chains, the level of that light chain would be increased and the ratio of the two

2/15/2018 KAPPA/LAMBDA LIGHT CHAIN		
Test Result	Mine	Normal
Free Kappa Lt Chain	2002 (VH)	3.3-19.4
Free Lambda Lt Chain	3.0 (L)	5.7-26.3
Kappa/Lambda Ratio	667 (VH)	.26-1.65

would be abnormal. As shown here, my kappa light chain results were very high, lambda light chains were low, and the ratio was very high; this was a strong indicator of multiple myeloma.

The complete blood count (CBC) measures levels of red cells, white cells, and platelets in the blood. If too many multiple myeloma cells are in the bone marrow, other blood cell levels can be low. Low red cells and low hemoglobin shown here were consistent with multiple myeloma.

2/14/2018 BLOOD CELL COUNTS		
Test Result	Mine	Normal
White cells	5.1	3.5-10.5
Red cells	3.94 (L)	4.30-5.70
Hemoglobin	12.6 (L)	13.5-17.5
Platelets	182	150-400

Throughout the day, I made several phone calls to Irma as medical teams met with me to report their findings. I enjoyed interacting with medical teams comprised of a top surgeon or physician, a resident physician, and student interns all working and learning together. This made me feel at home in an academic environment.

The neurosurgeon Dr. Coppens told me that I would need cranial surgery to remove the large mass pressing on my brain. I did not require emergency surgery but the tumor must be removed before it intruded further into the brain. Because the tumor shared blood vessels with the brain, this entanglement might add difficulty to the surgery.

Everyone was surprised that I had none of the symptoms expected from a large mass pressing on my brain: pain, vision problems, loss of feeling and mobility, digestive problems, etc. Many of us were thanking God that the tumor was identified so quickly and I had been spared these problems.

I called my two brothers and informed them about my condition. Of course they were surprised, but perhaps not greatly so. I was the first of us siblings to have a heart attack (November 2011) and now the first with cancer. I was beginning to see my life-threatening conditions as God's loving wake-up calls for all of us.

Friday, February 16, 2018

Dr. Coppens scheduled surgery for February 21 to remove the cancerous mass and cover the hole in my skull with an implant. This date allowed the doctor to order a custom implant. Before discharging me, my skull was scanned again specifically to measure for the prosthesis. The doctors talked about conducting more scans and bone tissue biopsies to assess the scope of my cancer and plan for future treatments, but a busy imaging schedule at the hospital and my desire to be at home convinced them to delay additional tests until I came back for surgery.

When I learned that I would be discharged on Friday, I called Irma to arrange a ride to get me. Because she and our son-in-law Josh arrived before I was officially discharged, both were present when two medical teams briefed us on my condition and the next steps. They were quite certain of the multiple myeloma diagnosis and the need for chemotherapy treatments following surgery.

This was the first time Irma remembers hearing the name, multiple myeloma. Josh promptly searched "multiple myeloma" on his phone and told Irma that the prognosis might be that I have 2 years to live.

I got home around 8 pm and communicated with the robotics team that I would be out for surgery and recovery. Sadly I would not travel with the Robo Raiders to Elgin, Illinois for the Illinois State FIRST® FTC Championship on February 23-24.

I knew that it was important to call for help from close friends in our church as we walked the uncertain path ahead. Although always hesitant to ask for help, I prepared an email that was sent to members of the church informing them of my situation and asking for prayer. I also asked Pastor Steve if the elders of the church would pray over us at their regular meeting Sunday morning.

Saturday, February 17, 2018

To prepare for my possible death, Irma and I reviewed our estate plan. We decided to revise beneficiaries for our retirement funds to better provide for Irma's needs and those of our many grandchildren.

Sunday, February 18, 2018

Irma and I went to church prior to the morning service to meet with the elders. They prayed over us and anointed me for God's healing according to James 5:14-15:

> "Is anyone among you sick? Let him call for the elders of the church, and let them pray over him, anointing him with oil in the name of the Lord. And the prayer of faith will save the sick, and the Lord will raise him up. And if he has committed sins, he will be forgiven."

After our time with the elders, Irma and I served as greeters because no one else was in place to do it. As we greeted arrivals, we received many hugs, offers of prayer for our uncertain journey, and offers of rides for Irma to St Louis and back.

That afternoon Irma and I enjoyed time together remembering God's goodness in years past and the help He provided us in times of trouble. We knew that our future was in the hands of a loving God who has power to make us strong when we are weak. We were thankful that even with a large tumor in my head, God had enabled me to feel completely normal, do things as any able-bodied person my age, and have great peace.

In the evening we attended a Bible study with our small group from church. We updated these friends on my upcoming surgery and mentioned Irma's needs for transportation because she was not comfortable driving in big city traffic. We received several offers of help for transportation or other needs. This support was an early taste of God's provision throughout the challenges ahead.

Upon returning home we got a phone call from Jim in Wheaton, Illinois, a friend from graduate student days at Cornell University. Jim was following up after my comment in January that our family may be in his area if the Robo Raiders qualified for the Illinois State FTC championship. Of course, I updated Jim on my health, my plans not to travel to Elgin, and current plans for Nancy and her kids to be at the robotics competition. Jim also inquired about details of the competition so he could take his grandson to watch. Jim also committed to pray for our needs.

Lastly, we called Doug and Mary Lou, pastor and wife in our former church in Pullman, Washington to tell them of my upcoming surgery and to learn from cancer struggles of their daughters. We received much encouragement, prayer, and offers to share our situation with others in their church for additional prayer support. God's web of support for our cancer journey was growing.

Monday, February 19, 2018

Irma and I had a phone call with Moody Bible Institute representatives to review current beneficiaries of our estate trust, which Moody administers. We learned how to make changes to our trust so it better fit our family and our perceived needs from this vantage point.

Tuesday, February 20, 2018

Irma and I called TIAA, who administers our retirement accounts, to get our trust beneficiaries revised to fit our desires. Janika, the representative with whom we spoke, helped us make changes and offered to have her church pray for us. We were beginning to see a huge prayer base behind us— family, friends, colleagues in work and ministry, and strangers across the nation. Our struggle would be fought from a position of supernatural strength.

Robo Raiders met at our home in the afternoon. I was able to participate fully and also began to prepare the team for my absence or limited involvements. Since we believed that God provided our home for ministry to others, I was able to confidently offer the Robo Raiders its use even if Irma and I were absent. I gave our grandson Thor (a member of Robo Raiders) a house key and instructions for providing access when proper supervision was present.

Reflecting on my upcoming surgery, it was interesting that neither Irma nor I had suspected that I had cancer. The lump on the back of my head had been unnoticed by Irma and simply an item of tactile interest to me. To get a better feel for the visual evidence of my cancer, I asked Irma to photograph my head from the side so I could compare its shape before surgery with that after surgery.

Cranial Surgery
Debulking a Tumor

Cranial surgery was a new experience for me. Yes, I had experienced a number of lesser surgeries in my 73 years, but surgery around my brain brought new levels of uncertainty and risk. This surgery would be an opportunity to prove my trust in God.

Wednesday, February 21, 2018

Surgery was one week after the first CT scan of my tumor. Nancy drove Irma and me to SLU Hospital for 7:00 am pre-surgery check-in and surgery at 9:15 am. In about 2 hours, the neurosurgery team opened a large flap at the back of my head, "de-bulked" the tumor, screwed in the implant, and closed the flap with "zillions" of staples. Dr. Coppens left a portion of the tumor that shared blood vessels with the brain because he felt it was risky and could be controlled by chemotherapy.

When I came out of anesthesia, I found myself in a general ICU room where Irma and Nancy could visit. Although groggy, I understood that surgery had gone well and I had lost a lot of blood. I received two units of blood plasma during surgery plus two each of plasma and platelets shortly afterward.

During recovery the medical team closely watched my blood counts and blood pressure to detect any infections that might occur. Through the night I had numerous blood draws and repeated questioning to monitor my blood counts and test my abilities (memory, pain, movements, sense of feeling, vision, etc.). Thankfully, I had no infections and remarkably low pain levels. My post-surgery "turban" head wrap is shown in the picture.

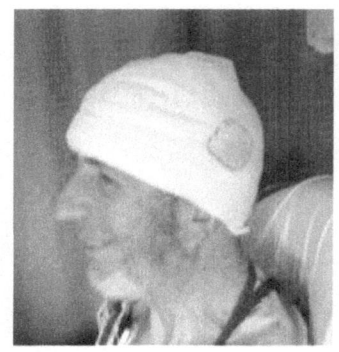

Thursday, February 22, 2018

On Thursday, Irma got a mid-morning ride from Sarah of our small group. Irma visited me in an ICU suite I shared with three patients suffering from brain or cancer-related problems.

Dr. Schoen a hematology oncology doctor took a bone core sample from my right hip away from suspected cancer lesions. The sample was sent for biopsy and genetic analysis. Biopsy results (see text box) showed 70% of cells in the bone marrow sample were myeloma. Multiple myeloma was clearly more widespread than just in my cranial tumor. Now I understood why doctors wanted to scan my body to identify "hot spots."

> 2/22/2018: BONE BIOPSY
> The bone marrow core biopsy is hypercellular for age and shows plasma cell myeloma (by CD138 immunohistochemistry, 70% plasma cells).

When my head wrap was removed, my bandage over the surgery site showed no wound bleeding. The surgical closure of my cranial opening and initial healing had gone well. That gave everyone some assurance that I would not be experiencing post-surgical bleeding.

About 3:30 pm Irma got a ride home from Brad, a friend from church who worked nearby. Later I heard that a full-body CT scan was planned to determine cancer activity throughout my body. I was moved to a peaceful single-person room where I had fewer interruptions, so I slept rather well for being in the hospital. I was now able to get up and walk, but I had a poor appetite and ate only what seemed to be tasty and moist.

Friday, February 23, 2018

I hoped to be discharged on Friday, but one of the surgeons was concerned that I might have lesions that required surgery or bracing to prevent bone breakage. They x-rayed me in many different places and from many orientations and found nothing of high risk for bone breakage. Medical personnel indicated that it was possible that I would be discharged Friday or Saturday, depending on whether I had more scans.

When my head bandage was removed, it revealed the extent of my head wound: from ear to ear. Thankfully there were no signs of post-surgery bleeding or infection. I had an inverted horseshoe of 67 staples along with blue markings, which Irma compared to the aligning of two pieces of fabric to be sewn together. (See photo). The wound did not cause me any pain so I was encouraged that all was going well.

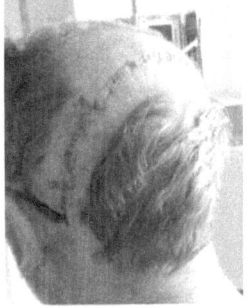

Irma and our oldest grandson Knut arrived at the hospital about mid-day on Friday. Knut had gotten home Thursday for quarter break at Rose-Hulman Institute of Technology. I doubt that either of them had thought about the scope of my surgery, so both were shocked at the size of my head wound. In our brief visit, I learned that Knut had done well both academically and personally in his second quarter. Being an engineer myself, I was very pleased to see his success as an engineering student at one of the top undergraduate engineering programs in the nation. After a short visit, Knut drove our car home and left Irma with me.

Gary, an elder from our church whose wife had travelled the cancer journey, visited us and shared their experiences dealing with cancer. As I listened to their story, I shuddered at the thought of cancer treatments, side effects, and the uncertainty of when cancer would return after it was beaten into remission.

That afternoon I was moved to a single room in the neurosurgery wing. While Irma was with me in my room, we recognized my nurse, John, as one who had served Irma seven months earlier when she was undergoing tests following her mini-stroke (cerebral amyloid angiopathy). John remembered Irma from the time she had been there.

At different times during the day I called my older brother Bob in Washington, Peter my colleague at Ohio State University, and Ralph and Connie in Idaho to inform them of my progress. I felt that I needed to keep people close to me informed about what was happening and how this might affect my capabilities in the future.

As it became clearer that I would be discharged, Irma and I had to find a ride home and clothes for me to wear. After a few calls, Josh gathered some clothes for me and brought them to the hospital. Irma and I shared my hospital dinner as we waited for Josh and my discharge. Because many departments were involved in my care, it took hours to get discharged. After I arrived home around 8 pm. I texted my younger brother Arnie to update him on my situation.

Saturday, February 24, 2018

I slept relatively well my first night at home. I had a good appetite but remained a bit low on energy. Pastor Steve visited Irma and me and encouraged us to watch the newly available livestreamed worship service at our church and to give him feedback. Laurie, wife of Kirk, a Mascoutah church pastor and friend of the family, brought us hearty chicken-rice-cheese soup that we really enjoyed.

I watched livestreamed FIRST® FTC Illinois State Championship robot matches much of Saturday. In division qualifier matches, the Robo Raiders placed #8 of 22. The Robo Raiders were the second pick by the #1 alliance, so they competed against other alliances in elimination and championship matches. Their alliance became the winning alliance for Illinois State, which qualified the Robo Raiders to advance to the North Super Regional Championship in Cedar Rapids, Iowa on March 15-17.

The Robo Raiders had performed well, but it appeared that they were really carried by their alliance partners to become part of the winning alliance. Their advancing to State was another example of God's kindness. I missed that I had not been present for this exciting experience for the team.

Sunday, February 25, 2018

I slept well going into Sunday. Irma and I stayed home from church and watched the morning service via livestream. Then we slowly walked around our block and hoped to see our family. To our delight, after their church service ended, Nancy and the children came bounding across Maple Park to pay a visit to "the sick". We shared a few hugs to celebrate my being able to get out and walk so soon after surgery. When I showed the family the stapled back side of my head, we saw shocked looks from many of the kids. But I was blessed to have so many of the family greet me.

I had naps on both sides of our Sunday lunch. That afternoon I began writing about my cancer experience to minimize errors in our memories that were already blurring. I also knew that I would need to remember what had happened so that I correctly reported progress to our many friends and relatives. I ended the day with my first bath and gentle hair wash since my surgery.

With successful and essentially pain-free surgery behind me, I was very thankful. God had wonderfully carried me through a serious medical procedure. I had vague ideas of chemotherapy treatments that might be ahead, but knew nothing of what I would actually experience. Again I knew that I must rely on the Lord to direct events and carry me through the challenges I would face.

Preparation for Chemo
Bracing for Change

Chemotherapy was completely new to me. I had known others who underwent chemo treatments but had never experienced it myself. I now had an opportunity to learn experientially what chemotherapy meant and feel how the patient felt throughout the process. I also could see how it affected the patient and loved ones around the patient.

Monday, February 26, 2018

On Monday, I had a post-operation appointment with Dr. Pritchett my primary care physician. He helped me identify Dr. Rodriguez at Illinois Oncology in nearby Swansea for my chemotherapy; we hoped this would negate a need for frequent travel to St Louis for chemo treatments. Dr. Pritchett wrote prescriptions for eye and nasal meds to stop apparent minor infections before I began chemotherapy.

Over the next few days I received many expressions of love and prayers from people in our church, co-workers, friends from the past, and Christians we encountered in our business interactions. I was greatly encouraged to know that many people were petitioning our great God and Savior who has power to heal and sustain us in difficult times.

Tuesday, February 27, 2018

The Robo Raiders met on Tuesday to debrief on their Illinois State Championship experience and plan for super regional competition. I was pleased that they saw the hand of God in their Illinois State success. I also took the opportunity to share how God had carried me through my surgery experience, and I showed them my head wound. This helped to remind all of us that success at NSR would also be in the hands of our Lord.

The team expressed a strong desire to be successful at FTC North Super Regionals (NSR) and advance to FTC World Championship in Detroit in late April. I helped them conduct a design review for their robot, which showed they had good potential for adding an effective retrieval system that could make them competitive at the NSR.

February 28-March 5, 2018

With chemo in the near future, I became increasingly health conscious. I felt a need to stay warm to avoid sickness, so I began wearing a jacket and cap to avoid chills when working in the garage. When I noticed pain in my right ribs, I wondered if this was related to multiple myeloma. Irma and I began thinking that I should start chemotherapy soon to ward off multiple myeloma spreading to other parts of my body.

I wondered if I should plan my usual professional travel since I did not know how cancer and chemotherapy treatments would affect me. Under consideration were the Capstone Design Conference in Rochester, New York in early June and the annual conference of the American Society for Engineering Education in late June in Salt Lake City, Utah. Both were important places for networking and promoting my work products. What would I be able to do by June? What should I trust God to enable me to do?

As Irma and I anticipated my deteriorating health, I strengthened my resolve to reduce potential impacts on Irma. I wanted to enclose our garden space to keep critters away from our crops and reduce the care needed for our garden. We also discussed converting my educational resources (workbooks and card decks) into books that could be sold and shipped via Amazon-linked services, rather than the current process in which we sold and shipped my products.

I worked diligently to enclose the garden and orchard. I created a garden-orchard plan to fit in the available space, and I prepared a list of materials needed. I got help from Josh, Knut and Thor to pull out semi-dwarf fruit trees, and I ordered dwarf trees to fill the space. I planned a hip roof design enclosure over blueberry bushes, tomatoes, and other low-growing garden crops and 10-ft flat roof design over fruit trees. I planned to build the hip-roof first to prove my construction methods before ordering supplies for the taller part over the fruit trees.

Tuesday, March 6, 2018

On March 6, Irma and I got rides from Gary and Ross to and from doctor appointments at SLU. We discussed with Drs. Goyal and Schoen a plan for 6 months of chemo treatments from Dr. Rodriguez in Swansea until my cancer was in remission and blood cell counts were normal. Then we would return to Dr. Goyal to determine next steps. The doctors felt that I might be a good candidate for a stem cell transplant. All of this sounded ominous.

Next we met with Dr. Coppens to remove, as I counted, 67 staples from the back of my head. Dr. Coppens said that healing of my external surgical wounds had progressed well, but he wanted another visit in a few weeks to see that internal healing was also going well.

Wednesday, March 7, 2018

On Wednesday Irma and I met with Dr. Rodriguez at Illinois Oncology to plan chemotherapy as directed by Dr. Goyal. Dr. Rodriguez set March 12 to start treatments that included an injection twice per week, a weekly pill, and a daily pill. We would complete three or four chemo cycles over 10 to 12 weeks, then measure protein levels to see how the myeloma had been reduced. Excessive protein production must be brought to normal levels so that my bone marrow could produce the red blood cells needed for energy and white cells for resistance to disease.

March 8-11, 2018

I pushed hard to make progress on several fronts prior to starting chemo. At the same time the Robo Raiders worked long hours to prepare for the North Super Regional championship.

Seeing that my chemo treatments would end in May and believing that my health would be good, I decided to attend the Capstone Design Conference in early June. There I could help Peter present a workshop and promote my books to my primary target audience. I decided not to attend the ASEE Conference in Salt Lake City due to distance and lesser benefits expected.

For my book publishing, I chose Create Space, a print-on-demand publisher that makes books available for sale through Amazon. I then converted card decks that I previously sold into two 6x9-inch books: *Teamwork Minutes* and *Design Thinking*.

Having good energy, I began serious garden preparation. I set up two 4x4 foot raised beds and planted asparagus seeds, lettuce, and spinach. I set up a trellis and planted snow peas and snap peas. I mulched leaves and set up another 4x8 foot raised bed in the enclosure.

I felt ready to begin chemotherapy. I had made significant progress on key responsibilities. Walking into the lion's den would have been scary without confidence in God.

Chemotherapy Phase 1
Dosing and Monitoring

Chemotherapy is filled with many uncertainties. How would drug combinations affect my cancer, mitigate side effects, and otherwise affect me? How effectively would monitoring determine effectiveness of treatments and detect any side effects that needed to be addressed? Would we wait weeks before knowing if treatments were working? Chemo would provide another opportunity to learn patience and to trust both medical professionals and God.

Monday, March 12, 2018

My chemotherapy began March 12, about one month after the cancer was detected. My regimen included three different treatments. Monday mornings I took 40 mg (10 pills, 4 mg each) of Decadron (Dexamethasone), a class of steroid hormone often used to treat multiple myeloma. This anti-inflammatory and anti-nausea treatment had some direct impacts on myeloma and minimized nausea from other treatments.

The afternoon of my first day, I went to Illinois Oncology for a Velcade injection. Velcade (bortezomib) blocks or slows action of proteasomes which break down proteins in both healthy and cancerous cells. Although I had feared that I would have a port installed for administering this drug, I received a simple injection in tissue under an arm. A blood sample was drawn weekly for lab analysis to determine the injection amount. I received a Velcade injection on Mondays and Thursdays over a two-week period, followed by a week in which I received no injection, then the cycle repeated.

My third treatment was a 25 mg Revlimid pill taken 21 successive days, taking none for a week, then repeating the cycle. Revlimid (lenalidomide) is a prescription medicine used to treat people with multiple myeloma (MM) in combination with dexamethasone, or as maintenance treatment after autologous hematopoietic stem cell transplantation. Because Revlimid has potential for genetic alteration, special approvals were required, and shipping came directly from an authorized pharmacy. I took a Revlimid pill each day at noon. Thankfully, a grant was approved to offset the very high cost of Revlimid.

I weathered my chemotherapy treatments with only minor discomfort and side effects. The Velcade injection was quick, relatively painless, and did not make my hair fall out as I had feared. I noticed that my taste buds were less sensitive and my lips occasionally felt a bit puffy. I had minor nasal drainage and minor nose sores at times. I experienced minor constipation. Most notable was a problem with my sleeping; I was unable to sleep very much the night after I took the Decadron pills, even when I took Melatonin or Benadryl.

During my first week of chemo I read that multiple myeloma patients are 15 times more likely to die from infections than is the normal population. This information brought to mind the warnings of Dr. Rodriguez that I need to stay away from people who are sick and little kids, who are germ factories. These concerns caused me to sanitize my hands frequently and I began wearing a face mask when going into places where many people were present.

Thursday, March 15, 2018

Thursday I planted a row of raspberries inside the garden enclosure. I hauled compost and prepared holes for 12 raspberry roots offered by Charles and Carolyn, friends from our small group. They arrived with lovely raspberry roots and (to my surprise) a load of compost, and Charles helped me plant the roots with generous amounts of compost. What a surprise and blessing!

When two dwarf peach trees arrived, I planted these and a cherry tree that had arrived earlier. I pruned the trees and applied a dormant spray to my fruit trees, blackberries, blueberries, and raspberries.

Today the Robo Raiders traveled without me to Cedar Rapids to compete in the FTC North Super Regional. Over the next 2.5 days, they presented before judges, interacted with the public, and competed in robot matches. They placed 6th of 36 teams in robot competitions, then they competed unsuccessfully in the division championship. The Robo Raiders team was recognized as the only team competing in this super regional five years in a row. They were judged the 3rd place winner of the Connect Award, recognizing their relationships with professionals in engineering. The Connect Award qualified them to advance to the FTC World. Wow! The Lord had blessed them again so they could continue up the competition ladder.

Sunday, March 18, 2018

March 18 was the 46th anniversary of Irma's and my wedding day. My health prevented us from doing much celebrating, not even going out for dinner. But we enjoyed recalling so many ways that God had blessed our 46 years together. Our covenant relationship ensured our love and enabled us to live openly without fear of rejection. I wore a medical mask to church and to our small group that evening because of my concerns about being susceptible to contracting diseases.

Monday, March 19, 2018

Monday began a series of events that emphasized to us the seriousness of my treatment regime. I began the day taking 10 pills at breakfast, not knowing that they were the wrong pills. I went for a walk with Irma but felt sluggish. During the day I had difficulty staying focused and napped a lot. Irma drove when I went for my weekly injection. That night I slept well.

Tuesday, March 20, 2018

Tuesday morning due to my drowsiness, I did not walk with Irma; instead I napped. Mid-morning Irma discovered that the previous day I had taken 10 anti-nausea (10 mg prochlorperazine) pills instead of 10 Decadron pills. When we realized our error, I took the 10 Decadron pills before lunch to make up for their absence in my regimen.

As the day progressed, my lips and tongue felt strange and showed swelling. Mid-afternoon Irma called Geri at Illinois Oncology, who instructed us to go to emergency at a hospital. Irma drove us to St Elizabeth's

Hospital where, after a very long wait, I received a steroid shot to counteract the anti-nausea overdose. We learned a lesson to double check medications before taking them.

That afternoon the Robo Raiders met in our home, so my sudden departure to the emergency room left them wondering. With the other mentors present, they were able to continue work as normal.

His Lighthouse ministry to boys met in our home that evening while Irma and I were at the hospital. From the emergency room, I asked Josh to oversee the evening's activities. As planned, Josh led construction activities for the boys, and another man taught the Bible lesson. Josh and others served refreshments that Irma had prepared. The men cleaned up afterwards. This showed that my multiple myeloma can disrupt plans and require others to step in.

Amazingly, God orchestrated events of these two days so that I was spared serious effects from my overdose and everything else continued as scheduled.

March 21-27, 2018

I worked to get *Design Reviews*, *Professional Teamwork Mentor*, *Teamwork Minutes*, and *Design Thinking* books ready with all supporting information online for print-on-demand through Create Space. I ordered a printed proof of *Professional Teamwork Mentor* to see the quality of the final product. After proofing, these four books were offered for sale on Amazon.com: https://goo.gl/ekRaiz

The last week of March I was busy working on my enclosure. I installed posts and a gate, setting boundaries for my enclosure. With the help of Thor and Bjorn, my grandsons, I began installing 1-inch hex fencing on top of the hip roof structure. I was gaining confidence that the enclosure could be completed as planned.

Wednesday, March 28, 2018

On March 28, I met with Dr. Gupta my cardiologist for an annual checkup; these began after my heart attack of November 2011. Based on lab results and blood pressure, Dr. Gupta stated that my heart appeared to be in good condition. When I told him about my multiple myeloma, he immediately said I needed ultrasound imaging of my heart to determine if excessive proteins had been deposited by the myeloma. A week later I had an echocardiogram which showed that my heart had no excessive protein deposits. That's what I expected, but I also thanked God for the good report.

Sunday, April 1, 2018

We celebrated Easter with Knut home from Rose-Hulman and Paige (Josh's sister) visiting the family. Because Paige was working in cancer research in Montana, we learned how new treatments are making their way into cancer therapies. This reinforced Dr. Goyal's statements about how rapidly cancer treatment is changing. We became more convinced that stem cell transplants that extend one's life increase the possibilities that new cures could extend life even further. We also reminded ourselves that God numbers our days, and He determines how each of us responds to a treatment.

Monday, April 2, 2018

Irma and I met with Dr. Rodriguez to review progress from the chemotherapy. As shown here, red cells and hemoglobin levels remained below normal levels, but they had improved from levels before chemotherapy began. Dr. Rodriguez said we would continue current treatments

4/2/2018 BLOOD CELL COUNTS		
Test Result	Mine	Normal
White cells	4.3	3.5-10.5
Red cells	3.42 (L)	4.30-5.70
Hemoglobin	10.7 (L)	13.5-17.5
Platelets	232	150-400

through May. When I told him of my plans to attend a conference in Rochester, New York the first week of June, he said we could stop treatments for my week of travel, then test protein levels to see if we needed to increase chemo dosages.

The Robo Raiders had a busy first week of April working on their robot and mentoring two less competitive teams from Kirkwood, Missouri. Being concerned about my low immunity to illness, during the mentoring session I wore a medical mask and stayed in the shadows most of the time.

April 2-14, 2018

The first week of April I found my business website, VerityDesignLearning.com, corrupted. I contacted Eric, my website developer in Ohio, for his help. We worked out a simpler website that would no longer make sales and handle transactions. I was now committed to making all sales through the Amazon listings and any promotions I accomplished by other means. This was a blessing to us in that I wanted to reduce the responsibility that Irma and I carried in managing my business.

The second week in April I got a full day of help from Knut working on my enclosure over the fruit trees. We built a 10-foot high structure to support fencing for the sides and fencing overhead. The next few days Irma helped me stretch hex-mesh fencing overhead for the enclosure roof.

During this period I wrote a 4-page paper, *Mighty Minutes for Professional Learning*, that I would present as a poster at the Capstone Design Conference. I drew from my experiences teaching and assessing student performance in team design projects and addressed the problem that students (and adults alike) do not like attention diverted from project work to develop stronger professional skills. My paper promoted frequent short professional topics discussions in teams for just-in-time infusions of professional skills to make project work more effective.

I also worked with Peter at OSU to develop an agenda for our workshop which had been approved for offering at the Capstone Design Conference. Although I was unsure about being able to attend the conference, I clearly wanted to contribute what I could while I could.

April 15-21, 2018

The third week of April I took steps to promote my books. I prepared a message to be shared with my contacts on LinkedIn. I described my four books and pointed people to my website and to their listings on Amazon.com. I got a response from Todd, a former graduate student at WSU, who spoke positively about these books and suggested that I write an article for LinkedIn.

I continued to be amazed that I was not experiencing weakness, pain, or other side effects of my chemotherapies. I spent time reading about these therapies to understand what I might expect in weeks to come. I found that stem cell transplants are becoming more common for multiple myeloma patients. I also learned about the transplant process and saw how greatly this might impact me for a number of weeks or months. But, for the time being, I needed to do as much as I could before things got worse.

April 22-30, 2018

During the fourth week of April, I prepared for the Capstone Design Conference. I prepared my poster and reserved lodging at the conference. I also researched travel destinations that could be scheduled before or after the conference: visits to friends in Ithaca, New York and visits to Irma's family in Ontario. I wanted to see people important to us before I experienced poorer health that prevented such visits. I was feeling great and confident that I could travel and participate in the conference.

Once I had committed to attending the Capstone Design Conference, I was asked by organizers to accept additional roles at the conference. The first was to moderate a panel discussion on new accreditation requirements for engineering degrees. Later I was asked to serve on two additional panels: one on team roles and the other on assessing professional skills in design projects. I accepted all of these invitations, again based on my hope of having good health the first week of June.

My oncology appointment on April 26 was the first day I did not wear a face mask for chemotherapy. When the treatment nurse commented on this, I told her that I had worn it because Dr. Rodriguez had "put the fear" in me when we started the chemotherapy. However, when I recently saw my white blood cell counts in the normal range, I felt that I could go without the mask. She agreed. This table shows that my white cell counts were normal but red cells and hemoglobin continued to be low.

4/23/2018 BLOOD CELL COUNTS		
Test Result	**Mine**	**Normal**
White cells	7.2	3.5-10.5
Red cells	**3.96 (L)**	4.30-5.70
Hemoglobin	**12.3 (L)**	13.5-17.5
Platelets	275	150-400

That week I continued covering the enclosure's hip roof with fencing and finished its gates. I periodically watched livestream matches of the Robo Raiders competing at FTC World in Detroit. The team's robot performed moderately well, and the team won the Connect Award, the first time they had ever won an award at the FTC World competition. I had missed being a part of the team's exciting finish to the season and I wondered what would be my involvement in the future.

May 1-5, 2018

During the first week of May, I worked hard to get the garden enclosure finished and ready to plant. I moved and rebuilt raised beds from previous years' gardening areas. I staked down fencing around the sides to keep animals from digging under it. I repaired holes in the fence and tied sections together to cover possible entry points. 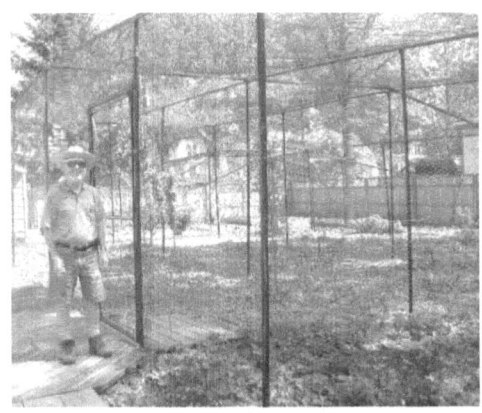 The day when I tied together overhead parts I overexposed my eyes to the sun, producing much watering and discomfort in my eyes. I learned to wear sunglasses when working outside. The photo shows my enclosure nearly completed.

Irma and I planned visits before and after the Capstone Design Conference. We set appointment times with friends in Ithaca, New York before the conference and with her siblings in Ontario, Canada after the conference. I also made lodging reservations for a 2-day drive to Ithaca and a 2-day return home through Ontario. Our trip was coming together to give us special personal visits if the Lord enabled me to travel well in June.

May 6-12, 2018

The second week in May I cleaned up around our property and built a trellis for blackberries in the enclosure. I built a raised bed for boysenberries and planted beans, zucchini, sweet corn, tomatoes, melon, and boysenberries. I dug up some old raspberry plants that survived the previous year's move and planted them inside the enclosure to complement the row Charles had provided. My garden plan was becoming more complete and much of it had been implemented. The final garden plan is shown. The aronia berries and strawberries lie outside the enclosure.

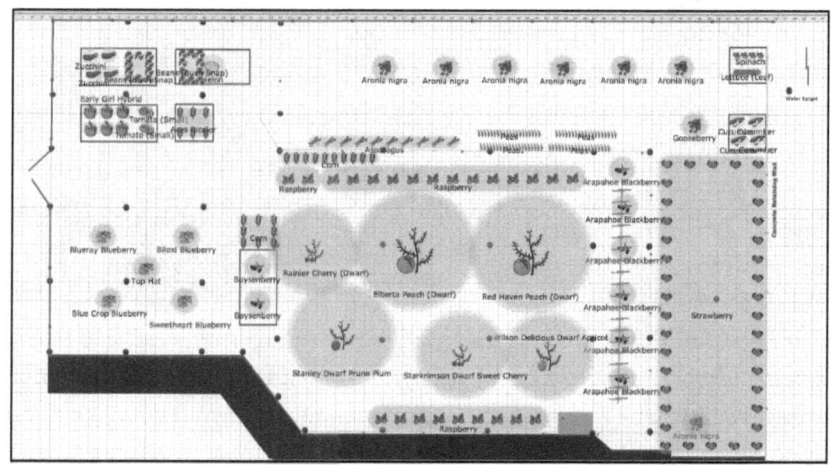

I continued to feel very good overall, but Irma noticed that my voice was affected by the chemo treatments. I felt some "thickness" in my mouth, and my teeth felt as if they were "on edge." I had minor sores in my nostrils, and my eyes tended to weep and stick shut over the night. Apart from these minor side effects, I felt perfectly normal! I had energy to continue a daily 3-mile walk with Irma after breakfast, and we often took a 5-mile bike ride after dinner. I was able to participate in family activities, but I stayed away from events with lots of people, especially lots of kids. I had energy to do physical work and clarity of mind to do work at my computer. God had blessed me with chemotherapy that did not take a huge toll on my life.

Sunday, May 13, 2018

On Mother's Day, Irma and I joined our family on our annual trip to the

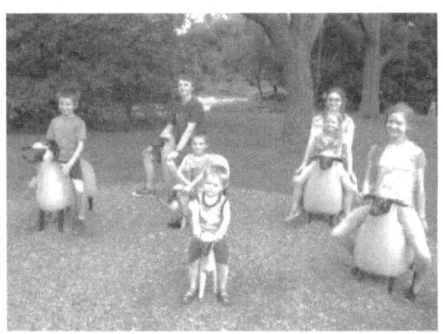

Missouri Botanical Gardens. It was a hot, sunny day, so I wore a straw hat and sun glasses for protection from the sun. Even in this hot and somewhat tiring outing, I did not suffer any health problems. The little kids found the best recourse for managing the heat: running through a fountain to cool off. I was pleased that all of our grandchildren were present, except Knut who was away at college. The photo shows our grandchildren, minus Knut and Sylvia, our oldest two.

While at the botanical garden, I took photos of family members to remember good times together before harder times came. I got photos of Irma and me (shown here), couples, and the whole family. We finished our

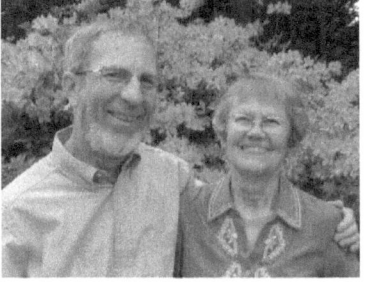

Mothers' Day celebration at a nearby nitro ice cream shop, Ices Plain and Fancy, where we devoured ice cream (mint chocolate chip for Irma and me) made from scratch right before your eyes.

Tuesday, May 15, 2018

On May 15, I drove to SLU Hospital for a CT scan of my head so Dr. Coppens could check internal healing. The scan showed desired healing. It did not show regrowth of the tumor, though the CT scan was not for that purpose.

My head felt normal apart from a numb feeling as I rubbed where the implant covered the hole in my skull. I wondered if my profile had changed. The photo shows the "after" profile (a dashed line) over the "before" profile of my head. The shape difference gives some indication of the bulge the tumor caused on the back of my head; it is puzzling that Irma had not noticed the bulge before I pointed it out.

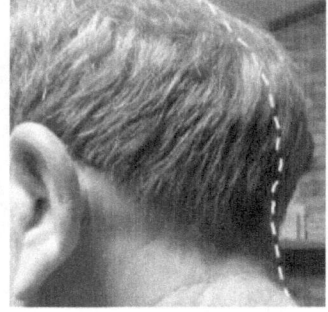

May 16-31, 2018

The remainder of May was used to prepare for our early June trip. I ordered my poster and Verity give-away bookmarks for the conference. Sadly, because I was avoiding crowds, I did not participate when the Robo Raiders represented FIRST® programs to information technology leaders at the Gateway to Innovation conference in St Louis.

In response to a request from the American Society for Engineering Education (ASEE), I wrote a brief history of my personal and professional life. ASEE wanted Fellow histories to show how varied paths can lead to recognition in the field of engineering education. The story of my heritage, education, work experience, professional accomplishments, and God's role in shaping my life is viewable at: http://ethw.org/First-Hand:ASEE_Fellows. Writing this personal history reminded me how God used people and opportunities to shape my life. Yes, God had done this in the past and would surely do so in my future with multiple myeloma.

Garden work demanded more time before our trip. With help from our grandkids, Irma and I picked strawberries, then Irma made jam. I planted more crops and applied pesticides to control insects in my garden.

June 1-3, 2018

We left home June 1 with our GPS acting weirdly and Irma feeling a bit strange. We began our trip anyway believing that God would enable us to complete the trip as planned. Friday we drove 12 hours, and Saturday we drove the remainder of the way to Ithaca.

Our first stop was to visit Ted, long-time friend and proprietor of White Church Cabin Country Store of many collectibles (shown here). Irma and I were able to poke around in his store and also lovingly view things his famed quilter wife Nancy (our daughter's namesake) left behind after her death.

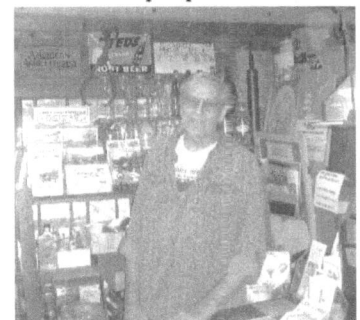

That evening we had supper with friends from years past: pastor Merold (who married us) and his wife Margaret; Don and Joan (match-makers for Irma and me); and Letty (influential in our Christian growth years ago).

Irma and I overnighted in Thomas Farm Bed & Breakfast, formerly a farmhouse where we lived the first year of our marriage. Sunday morning we attended Bethel Grove Bible Church, where we were married on March 18, 1972. We thanked God that my health enabled us to relive years past and reconnect with friends who had shaped our lives.

June 3-6, 2018

Sunday afternoon I drove to Rochester, checked us into our hotel, and drove to the Capstone Design Conference site at RIT. I helped Peter and Kaycee conduct a meeting with advisors for our National Science Foundation (NSF) project to develop assessments for student motivation in capstone projects.

I told a few colleagues there about my encounter with multiple myeloma. I was feeling in good health and was hopeful that I could participate fully in the conference. That night, however, Irma and I had difficulty sleeping, so I began the conference quite tired.

I participated fully in the conference. I attended sessions, helped Peter and Kaycee conduct a workshop, served on three panels, and presented my poster. I was pleased to find a number of people intrigued by my use of "Mighty Minutes" to bring professional skills into project classes. As the conference ended, I thanked God that I had the ability to engage fully in professional activities.

June 6-8, 2018

On Wednesday afternoon, I drove Irma and me to Niagara Falls, NY, where we stayed for the night. Thursday morning I drove us past Niagara Falls (Canada side) to admire its beauty, and continued on to Elmira, Ontario, where Irma's older sister Rita and her husband Vic live.

We enjoyed a lovely lunch with Rita and Vic plus Irma's younger sister Lydia, and their brother Walt. Of course, we discussed my multiple myeloma and how amazingly I was able to travel and engage in life. To me it was a rich blessing seeing relatives whom I love and whom I thought I may not see again if my health deteriorated.

That afternoon I drove via Sarnia to the US, then to Lansing, MI for the night. Sunday we conveniently stopped at Country Life Natural Foods to purchase 200 pounds of Wheat Montana flour and 27 pounds of natural peanut butter to replenish our and Nancy's pantries.

We safely completed a long adventure enabled by our God, even with multiple myeloma along! I had been off chemotherapy for over 10 days, and I saw no negative impacts. But I did wonder if the myeloma had been growing during the discontinuation of treatments.

Cancer Remission
Initial Success

Multiple myeloma is described as treatable but not curable. This suggests an enemy that retreats and waits for an opportunity to attack again. My rapid return to normal blood counts after chemotherapy began suggested that the cancer was having less effect on me than when it was discovered. But could this be an indication of treatment success? Here we needed to trust the medical professionals to read conditions and prescribe strategies that would keep this enemy away.

Monday, June 11, 2018

Back home after travels, I quickly resumed chemotherapy. On June 11, Irma and I met with Dr. Rodriguez to check on the state of my health. Blood cell counts (shown) from that day revealed that white and red cells and platelets were within normal ranges! And I had been off chemotherapy treatments for nearly two weeks!

6/11/2018 BLOOD COUNTS		
Test Result	**Mine**	**Normal**
White cells	4.4	3.5-10.5
Red cells	4.3	4.30-5.70
Hemoglobin	13.2 (L)	13.5-17.5
Platelets	225	150-400

I was hoping this meant I was cured and could end treatments, but Dr. Rodriguez prescribed round four of the same treatments as before. He authorized Revlimid, I got a Velcade injection, and I took Decadron pills that afternoon. More extensive lab tests were scheduled for June 21, upon which the next course of action would be determined. I was surprised to find that I slept well after taking Decadron that afternoon, but I had trouble sleeping the next night.

June 12-20, 2018

I promoted my design and professional skills books to attendees of the Capstone Design Conference by personal emails that pointed them to the Amazon.com link for my books: https://goo.gl/ekRaiz. I also sent emails to people who in the past had purchased or requested examination copies of my books.

I received information about a September 23-25 meeting of the advisory board for the Iron Range Engineering (IRE) program in Virginia, Minnesota. I had served on the board for 10 years as this award-winning project-based engineering program developed. I told the program director about my multiple myeloma and stated that I would attend if my health permitted. I expected that treatments ahead would impact my body, but God might wonderfully enable me to drive 1500 miles to attend.

I faced a number of troublesome situations in early summer. Squirrels got inside my garden enclosure, so I had to locate holes and repair them. Japanese beetles infested my garden and caused a lot of damage before I got them under control. Hot summer temperatures required frequent watering of garden and flowers. Flowers planted by our front sidewalk repeatedly disappeared (rabbits?). Our pool was inoperable and unusable until plumbing problems were at least partly fixed.

Irma reminded me that God's word instructs us to rejoice under all conditions. We need to trust that God is working all things together for our good (Romans 8:28):

> *We know that in all things God works for the good of those who love Him, who have been called according to His purposes.*

In response to Irma's recommendation, I began reading Randy Alcorn's book, *Heaven*. This book gave me a much better understanding of heaven and how God uses life experiences to prepare us for our future in heaven. Note that heaven is the destination of people who have listened to God and accepted what He says: Jesus is God's Son and must be Lord of our lives.

Jesus told His followers that He would go and prepare a place for them in heaven. This does not apply to people who are not His followers.

My greater understanding of heaven encouraged me as I faced uncertainty due to cancer. Yes, God was using cancer to work changes in my life that would better prepare me for heaven. This gave me reason to be joyful when things didn't seem to be going well. As stated at the beginning of this book (James 1:2-4, NKJV):

> "Count it all joy when you fall into various trials, knowing that the testing of your faith produces patience. But let patience have its perfect work, that you may be perfect and complete, lacking nothing."

June 21-30, 2018

Blood work done on June 21 measured several blood components, nearly all of which fell within normal limits. When we met with Dr. Rodriguez on June 25, he entered the examination room saying: "Congratulations, young man; results look good!" He described my test results as "fabulous" because key measures reached good levels in a 3-month period, when normally it took over 6 months. Wow! He suggested beginning an 8-week "maintenance" routine that would continue only the pills I had been taking, no shots. Subsequent test results would guide decisions on future treatments.

After this meeting, Dr. Rodriguez spoke with Dr. Goyal, my oncologist at St Louis University Hospital. She wanted to discuss the test results with us and decide next steps, which we assumed included stem cell transplant therapy. Irma and I remembered that earlier Dr. Rodriguez had described stem cell transplant as "horrendous". Dr. Goyal's office sent us a packet of information on stem cell transplants in preparation for a July 2 meeting.

Life challenges continued as we waited for the July 2 appointment. Inappropriate charges to my business website forced us to stop automatic payments. I also downgraded my website, which caused issues with website function. A severe thunderstorm passing through the area brought high winds, 3 inches of rain, a fruit tree blown over, and many downed limbs in our yard. We struggled to rejoice in God as we worked through these issues.

Monday, July 2, 2018

On July 2, Irma, Nancy, and I went to SLU's Blood and Marrow Transplant (BMT) clinic to meet with Dr. Goyal. Before the meeting, two nurses tapped both arms before obtaining 10 blood samples needed for pre-transplant tests. They said another 20 samples would be drawn another day to more fully check my eligibility for a transplant. Ouch!

Test results showed most of my conditions in normal ranges, but some barely. As shown, my white and red cells and platelets were within but near the lower ends of normal ranges. Light chain proteins were near normal conditions but the ratio of kappa to lambda portions was high.

7/2/2018 BLOOD COUNTS, LT CHAIN PROTEINS		
Test	Result	Normal
White cells	3.8	3.5-10.5
Red cells	4.33	4.30-5.70
Hemoglobin	12.7 (L)	13.5-17.5
Platelets	161	150-400
Free Kappa Lt Chains	19.4	3.33-19.4
Free Lambda Lt Chains	10.0	5.7-26.3
Ratio Kappa/Lambda	1.94 (H)	0.26-1.65

Dr. Goyal described my medical history and summarized considerations before a stem cell transplant decision:
- Blood cell counts and protein analysis showed multiple myeloma under control in a very short time.
- Genetic analysis showed that my multiple myeloma may come back more quickly than average.
- My good health suggested that I might respond better to treatments than many patients much younger than I.
- Stem cell transplant could greatly reduce cancer and delay its return 2 years longer than otherwise.
- Stem cell transplant would take about 2 months, including many tests prior to transplant and recovery.

We learned that the stem cell transplant process included:
1. Many tests to find any disqualifying illnesses or infections
2. Injections stimulating stem cell production and mobility
3. Apheresis to extract stem cells from my blood
4. High-dose chemotherapy to kill bone marrow and cancer

5. Infusion of my stem cells for growth in bone marrow
6. Marrow increasing blood counts and resistance to infections
7. Return to maintenance chemotherapy

Irma and I were surprised by the length of the treatment and recovery process. We had thought that the whole process might be 2-3 weeks, but that was the time from high-dose chemo to having acceptable blood cell counts. We were glad to have Nancy with us to help us grasp what was said.

We received a notebook that described the Blood and Marrow Transplant (BMT) Program and staff, autologous (using your own) stems cell transplant, screening process for eligibility, inpatient and outpatient transplant options, transplant phases, and support services.

A tentative timeline proposed for my autologous transplant, by week was:

July 23: Many tests and social evaluation
July 30: Discuss eligibility; make decision on transplant
August 3: Prepare and collect stem cells from me
August 15: Hi-dose chemo; infuse my stem cells
August 20: Recovery, restore blood count and strength

Irma and I discussed stem cell transplant and how it would affect us and our family. We considered its potential to extend my life, physical and emotional stress for Irma and me, Irma's transportation needs, and increased responsibilities for Irma and family in my absence. My thoughts gravitated to my primary responsibility: caring for my wife in her years ahead. Her mini-stroke last year revealed that she would be susceptible to strokes in the future. Our home, pool, and property were burdens beyond Irma's abilities to manage. I reasoned that a transplant adding years to my life would enable me to be a better caregiver for Irma.

We had been praying for wisdom. The Bible says (James 1:5):

> "If any of you lacks wisdom, let him ask of God, who gives to all liberally and without reproach, and it will be given to him."

As the family saw my reasoning for a transplant and believed they could handle the extra responsibilities, I sensed that the Lord had guided us to prepare for a transplant. The next day, I called the BMT program office and indicated my desire to proceed. I was comforted in that if God did not want the transplant to occur, I could yet be found ineligible for the transplant based on testing.

Transplant Decision
Start Anew?

I had been told earlier by Dr. Rodriguez that stem cell transplant was a "horrendous" experience. In contrast, I was told by SLU BMT doctors that they regularly conduct successful transplants that add years to one's life. I also knew that undergoing a transplant would affect not only me, but also my family and others in our lives. Would the extensive tests that I had waiting shed needed light on the best decision?

Thursday, July 19, 2018

When I agreed to proceed with transplant preparation, the BMT staff arranged two days of tests for my eligibility. On July 19 I dropped off my 24-hour urine harvest and proceeded to a PET scan. Two different nurses tried putting an IV in two different arms before they succeeded and injected a radioactive sugar solution. The PET scan would highlight areas of high metabolic activity (cancer or infections) where the sugar solution had gone.

Next I got a chest x-ray which was uneventful. Then it took several tries and maintenance before they completed a Panorex scan of my mouth. I got an EKG while waiting for repairs on the Panorex machine.

After lunch Irma and I returned to the BMT clinic where nurses drew 20 samples of my blood after struggles of low flow rates from the IV. After the blood draws, Laura took a pencil-lead-sized bone marrow sample from my left hip for biopsy to measure the cancer cell presence in my bone. Then I drove us home.

Friday, July 20, 2018

Friday morning Irma and I followed the family on a visit to the St Louis art museum in Forest Park. We enjoyed free exhibits that interested us and the grandkids. We then picnicked before we returned home and the family drove to a wedding hours away. When we got home, Joe came to load the robot for an FTC scrimmage on Saturday near Chicago, where he and Knut would compete with a robot they had built over the summer. Yes, life was busy apart from dealing with multiple myeloma.

Tuesday, July 24, 2018

July 24 I had a second round of tests at SLUH. My day started with a glitch: I was given a wrist band that belonged to another patient. After I returned to the registration area for the correct wrist band, I wondered what would have happened if I had not paid attention to the wrist band. Thank you, Lord, for protecting me.

A MUGA test was conducted to measure the percentage of blood in my heart pumped out with each beat. A sample of my blood was made radioactive then returned into my body before X-ray images were taken to calculate the volume pumped. My left ventricle pumping percentage was 53%, just below the normal range of 55% to 70%, but above 50% required for the transplant. I wondered if the below normal performance was a result of my heart attack in 2011 that reportedly reduced my heart effectiveness by 15%.

Pulmonary function tests (PFT) measured my lung performance under different conditions. Although breathing in varied ways against different resistances was challenging, it was fun and educational because the PFT technician kept explaining to a medical student what he was doing, observing, and why. My performance was very strong for a person of age 73. Next I was asked to walk a marked route as far as possible in 6 minutes. When the technician told me part way through that I might be breaking the record for distance, I was motivated to walk even faster. In all, I was very encouraged by my stamina.

Over lunch, pre-transplant nurse Amber explained the transplant process to Irma, Nancy, and me. We were shocked at the duration and safeguards in the process. I would need 24-hour monitoring after high-dose chemo to detect undesirable reactions to treatments or infection. I would probably lose my hair and be very weak for about a week, starting 5 days after receiving my stem cells.

I would be admitted to the hospital (inpatient) when high-dose chemotherapy began. After my stem cell transplant, I could be an outpatient, making daily trips to the clinic and any emergency trips needed. We were greatly concerned about required isolation, monitoring, and daily travel the BMT clinic if I was an outpatient; this would place heavy burdens on Irma and Nancy.

The final test of the day was a fibroscan to look at liver function. The technician struggled to get good data from ultrasonic scanning, but finally the test worked and I was done in a few minutes.

When tests were over, Irma and I ate a snack in the sunshine and I drove us home. We had a lot to think about. We were concerned about impacts of high-dose chemo on my body. We also had concerns about travel from home to the hospital on a daily basis since Irma did not drive in St Louis traffic. The duration of my treatments in a given day would be unknown until test results for the day were available, making it very difficult to plan rides for us when I was not allowed to drive. It seemed that inpatient care was our best option from the start of high-dose chemo until my worst physical state was past; this might mean 2 weeks in the hospital.

July 25-29, 2018

With the potential of a stem cell transplant looming, I felt a need to get things done at home. Irma and I picked tomatoes, cucumbers, and blueberries and shared them with Nancy and neighbors. I enjoyed seeing God bless my garden and my being able to share its fruits with family and neighbors.

I staked up a butterfly bush and hibiscus plant, sprayed Roundup to kill grass around these plants, fixed gate and door functions, built a trellis for raspberries, added height to a blackberry trellis, and pruned fruit trees for more compact shapes. These improvements helped make the orchard and berry plantings easier to manage.

I checked online postings of test results as they became available. I did not find results for the PET scan (MUGA) or the bone biopsy so I called Laura to ask about these tests. She told me that my tests indicated that I would be eligible for a transplant. The MUGA scan showed no new sites with cancer, and the bone biopsy showed 0% cancer! Wow! Had God healed me of multiple myeloma? I was eager to hear Dr. Goyal's perspectives on Monday.

Monday, July 30, 2018

On Monday, Irma and I met with Dr. Goyal and Laura. Dr. Goyal discussed the test results and stated that my cancer was in remission. No infections or organ diseases had made me ineligible for a transplant. No new cancer sites were identified. My blood counts were in normal ranges. My light chain proteins were good but not quite in balance as they should be, so multiple myeloma might not be completely under control.

Dr. Goyal recommended that we proceed with the stem cell transplant. My good health and positive response to earlier chemotherapies suggested that my body could weather the transplant better than many others my age. Using my test data and histories of multiple myeloma patients receiving stem cell transplants, Dr. Goyal predicted that a stem cell transplant would give me four added years before my multiple myeloma came out of remission.

Dr. Goyal explained the process and timeline for my stem cell transplant. She explained what I would experience, risks along the way, and the many precautions their staff would take to prevent or control any problems that might occur. We discussed inpatient and outpatient options for the transplant process. In the end, Dr. Goyal pointed out that we had three options for handling incurable multiple myeloma: do nothing to treat it, resume maintenance chemotherapy treatments, or undergo a stem cell transplant followed by maintenance chemotherapy. Options, in this order, had greater lifespans predicted.

I signed my approval to proceed with the stem cell transplant process. That evening we had dinner with Josh and Nancy and with Sylvia (our oldest granddaughter) and her husband John. After dinner we discussed the transplant preparation, infusion, and recovery schedule and planned transportation for the early steps. The die was cast. Now we had to prepare for the emotional and physical trauma associated with the transplant.

Harvesting Stem Cells
Doing Blood Separations

In autologous stem cell transplants, stem cells are harvested from the blood plasma of the transplant recipient. With a stem cell infusion date of August 17, my stem cells were scheduled to be harvested on August 7 and maybe extra days if the harvest was inadequate in one day. The BMT staff planned to collect and freeze enough of my stem cells to enable two transplants.

Friday, August 3, 2018

I arrived at the BMT center with some trepidation, not knowing exactly what to expect. After being weighed (134 lbs), Colleen took a blood sample for a baseline from which to track my blood counts during the treatments. Blood counts posted later in the day are shown. My white cells had increased from the last test, red cells and hemoglobin had both fallen below normal levels, and platelets had slipped but remained in the normal range.

8/3/2018 BLOOD CELL COUNTS		
Test Result	**Mine**	**Normal**
White cells	5.2	3.5-10.5
Red cells	**4.26 (L)**	4.30-5.70
Hemoglobin	**12.9 (L)**	13.5-17.5
Platelets	174	150-400

In preparation for stem cell collection, I received my first injection of Neupogen (Filgrastim), a human granulocyte colony-stimulating factor that stimulates stem cell production. Although I had read that Neupogen injections can be painful, I felt very little pain. I was told that bone pain from the Neupogen injections may come later as the bones shift into high production.

A second preparatory step for transplant was installing a central line catheter for use in delivering chemotherapies, extracting stem cells, infusing stem cells, taking blood samples, or giving transfusions or other treatments. A central line tunneled venous catheter, or Hickman catheter, was prescribed.

Because staff gave me a mild sedative to relax me during the line installation, I was able to listen to step-by-step discussions of the surgical procedure. The surgeon used ultrasound guidance, a micropuncture needle, and microfilament wire to penetrate the right jugular vein and guide placement of the Hickman device. A metal tunneling device was used to penetrate the chest wall and prepare a path under the skin to guide the tri-fusion Hickman catheter to the jugular vein. Tunneling put distance between chest penetration and vein puncture, thereby reducing chances of infection. The catheter was sutured to the chest wall. The photo shows the three ports of the catheter following this procedure. I was shocked to see three ports dangling from my chest (as shown).

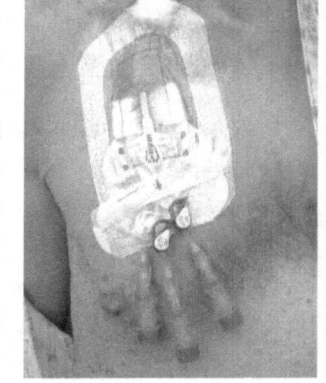

I had no serious discomfort from installation of the catheter or from its presence over the next several hours. But it was inconvenient trying not to put pressure on the device or lie on it at night.

Saturday, August 4, 2018

I received the second Neupogen injection on Saturday. Irma drove both ways to learn the route and test her confidence to drive to the hospital. I was given the injection and experienced very little pain. I was thankful that to-date this preparation for stem cell transplant had not been a painful process.

Sunday, August 5, 2018

Irma and I met early Sunday with the elders of our church so they could pray for me in preparation for the stem cell transplant process. Irma drove us to the SLU hospital for my third Neupogen injection and back again.

At the BMT clinic the nurse checked the dressing around my central line; a spot of blood I had seen was nothing to concern us. I received a Neupogen injection under my arm again with hardly noticeable pain. When I mentioned to the nurse that I had experienced no bone pain from these injections, she indicated that bone pain would not occur in all patients. I was thankful to have been spared this pain.

Monday, August 6, 2018

The fourth Neupogen injection was my transition to harvesting stem cells. At the BMT clinic I received the Neupogen injection, then a blood sample was taken from the central line (yay! no IV) to check if I was ready for stem cell collection and to establish baseline levels for cell counts.

As shown, all of my blood counts were outside of normal ranges, apparently affected by Neupogen injections I received. Most noticeably, white cells were much above the normal range, which was expected when stem cell production is being pushed. Other counts were marginally low but judged acceptable for stem cell collection to

8/6/2018 BLOOD CELL COUNTS		
Test Result	Mine	Normal
White cells	25.4 (H)	3.5-10.5
Red cells	3.96 (L)	4.30-5.70
Hemoglobin	12.5 (L)	13.5-17.5
Platelets	145 (L)	150-400

begin. Thus, I was instructed to return at 4:30 pm for a Mozobil (Plerixafor) injection. Mozobil is an immunostimulant used to mobilize hematopoietic stem cells in cancer patients and make them available for collection.

With time to kill before the Mozobil injection, Irma and I went to the St Louis zoo. Because the day was hot, we visited animals in shaded areas, indoor exhibits, and the butterfly house. We returned to the BMT clinic where I got the Mozobil injection then waited 30 minutes to be sure I did not have any reactions. On the way home, we got Chinese take-out to share with Josh and Nancy and their family. This gave us a wonderful time to report on my health status and arrange for transportation the next day.

Tuesday, August 7, 2018

August 7 was the first day of apheresis. In apheresis, blood plasma is removed from my body, it is separated into plasma and cells, my stem cells are collected, and remaining blood is returned to my body. Nancy drove me to the BMT clinic for 6:45 am check-in, then returned home. I received another Neupogen injection, and lab tests were done to characterize my blood before apheresis began.

Dr. Babic, the collections director, prescribed the blood flow rate based on my blood tests and set collection from 8:30 am until 1:30 pm. Mary closely monitored the process and made adjustments so that the collection was optimal as my blood was centrifuged to separate components. By noon Dr. Babic judged that the day's collection would not yield the 4 to 6 million cells desired, so he extended collection a half hour.

Collection ended at 2:00 pm. We waited for a cell count before knowing if I had to return for a second day of collection. About 5 pm, Stephanie from BMT came to announce the final count: 4 million stem cells collected. The decision from Drs. Babic and Goyal was that I needed a second day of apheresis, so I received a Mozobil injection to ready stem cells for collection in the morning. My granddaughter Sylvia drove us home.

I was pleased that collection went smoothly and painlessly. Having a good first day's collection, we expected that a second day of collection would meet our goal. This removed uncertainty in planning the rides I would need. I was delighted that I had experienced no distress from the process. I also came to appreciate the meticulous sanitation and quality control measures used in apheresis.

Wednesday, August 8, 2018

On August 8, I got a ride to the BMT with Nancy and her kids heading for a camping trip in Colorado. I arrived at 6:55 am, got a Neupogen injection, and gave blood for tests to guide the apheresis process that day. I sent this picture to Irma to show how I was lounging and enjoying my relaxing apheresis resort vacation.

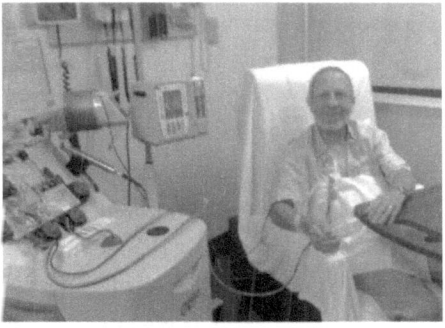

Day 2 of apheresis ended at 1:30 pm. Post-apheresis blood tests showed changes in my blood counts from those prior to apheresis. My white cells had increased, red cells and hemoglobin decreased, and platelets dropped much below normal levels. I was told that white cells would come down in the next few days. My very low platelet count meant that I must avoid cuts and bruises.

8/3/2018 BLOOD CELL COUNTS		
Test	Mine	Normal
White cells	**26.8 (H)**	3.5-10.5
Red cells	**3.49 (L)**	4.30-5.70
Hemoglobin	**11.0 (L)**	13.5-17.5
Platelets	**63 (VL)**	150-400

I was allowed to leave around 2:30 pm. I caught a ride home with Josh who had been purchasing building materials in the area. I did not know the day's stem cell yield until that evening when Stephanie called to report 2.5 million cells on day 2, yielding over 6.5 million cells for my use. That was enough!

That evening I realized again how God was watching over me. I entered this stage of treatment not knowing how I would feel during apheresis, the number of days required, the number of stem cells harvested, or how transportation would work out, but everything worked out very well. The skill and kindness of staff made the experience interesting and enjoyable.

I was reminded of God's blessings on my health overall when a staff member told that I looked 60, not 73. My multiple myeloma treatment experience to-date was much better than I had feared. Would this continue?

August 9-14, 2018

I had a few days at home to rest and prepare for the transplant process. I felt fairly normal but was frequently reminded that I had three ports hanging from my chest. I prepared an update on my health to email to family and friends to avoid making individual calls. To add a bit of humor, I spoke of my "apheresis resort vacation" and my bangles that were a poor attempt at body jewelry. I mentioned both my delight in God's provision and my trust in Him as we faced difficult treatments ahead.

I was feeling good; however, I had left garden and yard work to Irma, which made me feel guilty. One morning while I was working at my desk and Irma was harvesting tomatoes, I heard rapid footsteps and a shriek outside. Irma had been attacked by hornets where she was picking tomatoes. She got a number of painful stings, but thankfully she did not require medical attention. I got help from a beekeeper who identified a nest of ground hornets and helped us get rid of them.

In my week of waiting, I struggled a bit with sleep. I woke frequently with concerns about my central line; more than once I had broken into a sweat for a short time. Trying different sleep strategies did not resolve my problems. I finally called the BMT clinic and described my symptoms to Laura. She indicated that I should not be concerned about these conditions because I did not have a fever.

I also experienced swelling of my feet and ankles. When I called Laura, she indicated that the large amount of calcium infusion I received during apheresis would upset my body chemistry and could cause swelling. She said that this problem should disappear in a day or two. These experiences showed me that I did have side effects, but they were much less severe than I had imagined.

Irma and I received many words of encouragement from conversations, emails, phone calls, and mail. Local people offered rides and help. Friends from across the country (and out of country) offered prayers. We were told about God's care for us, His comfort, and the hope we have in

Him. People did not talk about blind luck that things would work out; we were reminded of God's promises that are certain to be fulfilled in times of smooth sailing and rough times. Yes, we needed this kind of preparation for the high-dose chemotherapy, stem cell infusion, and recovery ahead.

The myeloma drama had been playing out for several weeks, and perhaps the hardest part was just ahead. The timeline shown here gave me perspective on the current events but also reminded me that the end may stretch far beyond the timeline shown. I believed that God was not yet finished with me, because He was making me better prepared for eternity with Him.

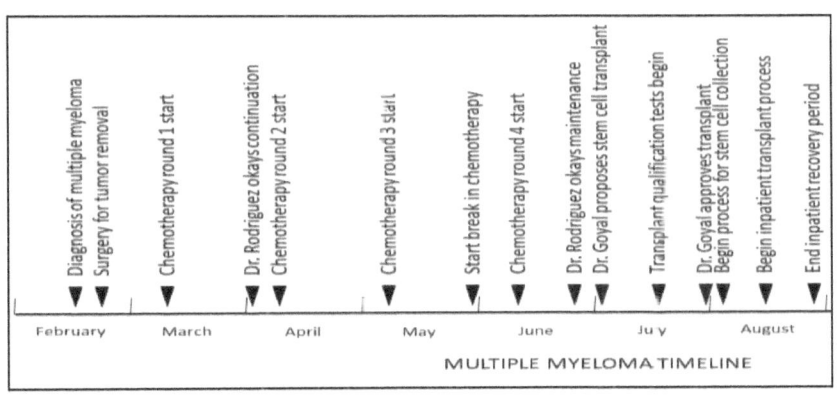

MULTIPLE MYELOMA TIMELINE

Stem Cell Transplant
Planting Blood Seeds

The most disconcerting part of the stem cell transplant process was high-dose chemotherapy that would kill bone marrow and blood cells. Side effects might include nausea, hair loss, and sores in mouth and gastrointestinal tract. I would experience weakness and loss of immunity after stem cells were infused into my body on Transplant Day 0.

As I approached high-dose chemotherapy, I held to God's promise (Isaiah 41:10):

> *Do not fear for I am with you; do not be dismayed for I am your God. I will strengthen you and help you; I will uphold you with My righteous right hand.*

Wednesday, August 15, 2018 (Transplant Day -2)

Cyndi (of our small group) drove Irma and me to the BMT clinic for the first day of chemo. After blood draws, Dr. Fesler explained the chemo process and obtained my written consent to proceed. He told me I would get a daily dose of 70 mg/m^2, lower than 100 mg/m^2 prescribed for younger patients. Before the chemo infusion, I was given antibiotic, antiviral, and antifungal medications to stave off potential infections.

Colleen explained the Transplant Day -2 chemotherapy schedule and wrote it on a whiteboard for Irma and my benefit:

Time	Steps
11:00 to 12:00	IV fluids to hydrate, prepare my kidneys
11:30 to 12:00	Anti-nausea triple treatment

11:50 to 1:30	Cryotherapy to prevent mouth sores
12:00 to 12:30	Chemotherapy to kill cancer cells
12:30 to 1:30	IV fluids to flush chemo from kidneys

The IV saline drip began an hour before chemotherapy started, paused during chemo, and resumed after chemo. This drip hydrated me and flushed my kidneys of chemo.

To avoid nausea and vomiting, I received a Fosaprepitant (Emend) and Palonosetron (Aloxi) drip and 8 mg of Dex (Dexamethasone) in pill form. We wondered if the Dex would produce insomnia as did a 40 mg dose I had taken weeks earlier.

I performed my own cryotherapy (see photo) by steadily sucking on ice to decrease blood flow (and hopefully chemo flow) to my mouth, thereby reducing potential mouth sores. Cryotherapy for 1 hour and 40 minutes chilled my body, so part way through it Irma wrapped me in blankets and fed me the snow cones. I did not find cryotherapy at all difficult or uncomfortable.

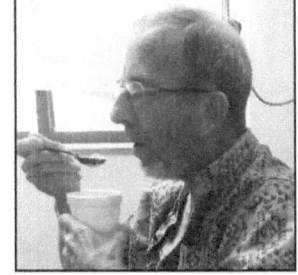

Melphalan, my high-dose chemotherapy, was infused for 30 minutes. Special precautions of staff showed the hazardous nature of this poison. The infusion went very smoothly. I learned that chemo would cause my blood cell counts to drop over the next few days. I was hopeful that the "low" dosage might lessen common side effects.

After chemotherapy, Colleen took me to the 8th floor north wing of the hospital and I was admitted. We had chosen inpatient care during the difficult part of the transplant process, so I was prepared to stay in the hospital a while. Irma helped me unpack, I set up my laptop, and I put on the wall Bible verses I had selected to reassure me of God's love and care. The hospital chaplain stopped by and offered his services 24/7.

My RN Shalu told us that all medications taken in the hospital must be provided by the hospital, so Irma gathered my bagful of meds to take home. We were shown the snack room and the small exercise room with a stationary bike. I was encouraged to be very active the first few days of my stay before I hit my lowest energy in a week.

Irma got a ride home provided by Ross from church. Nurses told me about my schedule, medications, and expectations. They recorded my vital signs on an 8-hour schedule and took blood samples at midnight so results were available to daytime staff on arrival. I felt very normal. I ate a full dinner and enjoyed it. I called Irma for a chat and to study the Scriptures and pray together. I was off to a good start. Thank you, Lord!

Thursday, August 16, 2018 (Transplant Day -1)

At 6 am I got up and dressed. I read from my Bible, prayed, and sang a few familiar Scripture songs. I enjoyed a big breakfast.

My transplant nurse practitioner Dan explained the transplant process, medications, and expectations for the next 2 weeks. Melphalan would attack cancer (and other) cells very quickly; cells would stop their activity and die in a few days. I would receive my stem cells (transplant) on Transplant Day 0, from which other events were referenced. Melphalan-caused drops in cell counts would produce neutropenia, abnormally few neutrophils in the blood, about Transplant Day +5. While neutropenic, I would be very susceptible to infection. During this time I would need isolation from possible infections until the stem cells had rebuilt my neutrophil absolute value to about 1000 (or 1.0 in my tables).

Shalu gave me meds, which included antiviral, antifungal, and antacid pills. The night's test results (shown here) indicate that Melphalan had brought red cells and hemoglobin below normal levels, but not dangerously so. When my hemoglobin or platelets might reach critical levels in a few days, I would receive transfusions to keep me alive and to prevent serious bleeding, respectively. The absolute neutrophil level, the best measure of infection fighting ability, looked good after 1 day of Melphalan.

8/16/2018 BLOOD COUNTS, ETC.		
Test Result	**Mine**	**Normal**
White cells	6.3	3.5-10.5
Red cells	**3.55 (L)**	4.30-5.70
Hemoglobin	**11.2 (L)**	13.5-17.5
Platelets	165	150-400
Neutrophil Abs	5.92	1.6-7.0

As done the day before, cryotherapy and hydration preceded the Day -1 Melphalan infusion. Dr. Rajeh and his transplant team checked my readiness for the day and answered questions. My cryotherapy started at 10:50 am and the 30-minute Melphalan infusion started at 11:20. After the infusion, I got more IV fluids and I continued cryotherapy until 12:50, when the high-dose chemotherapy process was declared finished.

My plan to take a nap and get some exercise was interrupted for taking vital signs and physical therapy instruction. Because chemo and inactivity could cause muscles to atrophy, I was given 10 exercises to do daily, in addition to walking. Although I didn't like being told I needed to do exercises, I was thankful that the hospital was looking out for my overall health. I also was told that I needed to drink lots of water to flush my kidneys of damaged stem cells.

Before night shift started, my nurse practitioner Megan prepared me for the next day's stem cell transplant. She said I would go through a "tenuous" state as my immune system bottomed out. I should expect a fever and other side effects that would need immediate attention to ensure my safety. Seeing my laptop open, she asked me what I was working on. I told her I was writing my multiple myeloma story (i.e., this book) to show others how MM impacts a life. She encouraged me to write it and asked to see it when it was finished. That was indeed encouraging to me!

Friday, August 17, 2018 (Transplant Day 0)

Many multiple myeloma patients call transplant day (Day 0) the turning point in their treatment: infused stem cells start rebuilding healthy blood. My nurse practitioner Dan and others prepared me and my room. I also received anti-nausea, antibacterial, and other medications for the day. Scripture verses posted in my room were read and used to encourage other staff struggling with personal issues.

My blood counts (shown here) indicated that I had not yet been affected much by Melphalan. White cells were in the normal range and slightly up from the day before. My absolute neutrophil score was high, further showing that my resistance to infection was good. Red

8/17/2018 BLOOD COUNTS, ETC.		
Test Result	**Mine**	**Normal**
White cells	8.9	3.5-10.5
Red cells	**3.4 (L)**	4.30-5.70
Hemoglobin	**10.6 (L)**	13.5-17.5
Platelets	174	150-400
Neutrophil Abs	**8.3 (H)**	1.6-7.0

cells and hemoglobin were slightly lower, but not greatly so. Platelets remained within the normal range. Dr. Rajeh told me that my good physical condition should help me respond well to the treatments.

About 11:30 am I was hooked to a saline drip. Next I took Tylenol and Benadryl pills to prevent my body from reacting to preservatives in the stem cells. Dan and Rachel started the transplant process at 1 pm and infused 5 bags of stem cells over the next hour. Each bag was thawed in a water bath just before infusion. My body did not react noticeably to the transplant, but I consumed one strawberry lollipop to help cover throat irritation expected during the process. (See photo).

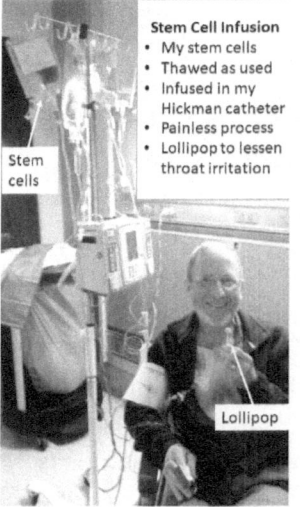

Stem Cell Infusion
- My stem cells
- Thawed as used
- Infused in my Hickman catheter
- Painless process
- Lollipop to lessen throat irritation

Stem cells

Lollipop

Because the transplant was a major milestone in my treatment, I marked its completion by striking a small gong that Dan had brought. After the transplant, I received more saline solution for about an hour to flush my kidneys of the stem cell preservative and any damaged stem cells.

I was told that the median time for stem cells to engraft into bone marrow was 11 days. Engraft in this case means that the stem cells are able to maintain an absolute neutrophil level of $5.0 \times 10^3/\mu L$ (i.e., 5000 per microLiter). When I reached this point, I could be transferred to outpatient care, assuming that I had no dangerous infections or other concerns.

After the stem cell transplant was completed, I took a nap, went for a walk, completed my exercises once more, and rode a stationary bike for exercise. Since staying active is part of a strong recovery process, I attempted to get all the exercise I could. At the end of the day shift, the nurse practitioner said I was being a model patient. Thank you, Lord, that I was able to be active so far.

During the night shift, RN Nancy checked my vitals on 8-hour intervals and drew blood at midnight. I appreciated these dedicated night staff who worked in poorly lit conditions, tried not to bother sleep-deprived patients, struggled with their own tiredness, and often had to respond to urgent needs that arose.

Saturday, August 18, 2018 (Transplant Day +1)

The day after my transplant I took an early walk in the hallway and overheard staff comment on the aroma of a transplant patient. Yes, today people smelled the fragrance of the preservative used in storing stem cells. I did my walking and stretching exercises anyway.

Both Laura and Dr. Rajeh encouraged me by explaining that my immunity remains strong, and the lack of observable symptoms indicates that the transplant is going well. They added to my pill diet one to prevent bacterial infections that may come as my resistance drops. They clarified my timeline: Day +10 transfer to outpatient, Day +30 transfer to Dr. Rodriguez nearer to home. I was concerned because outpatient required driving to BMT multiple times per week and I could not drive yet.

I learned from Laura that my case of multiple myeloma was much milder than those of most patients they saw. Most were diagnosed after MM had invaded their bones or organs causing intense pain, and often producing unprovoked broken bones. Thank you, Lord, my multiple myeloma was detected early and it had responded well to chemotherapy.

When Dr. Rajeh noticed my laptop open with my treatment update report in full view, he said, 'And what can we do to make your stay more enjoyable?" Laura chimed in with references to a hot tub and sauna being available. Then Dr. Rajeh added that he was just trying to get a good report in my update. I really appreciated how personable and helpful the staff had been.

I was somewhat discouraged by the looooooong treatment period expected after transplant. I assumed that I would not be able to travel to Minnesota for the IRE Advisory Board meeting in late September or to Ontario for a likely family reunion in early October. I would not be able to do yard work for the remainder of this season. I would not be able to drive for 30 days. But I was encouraged by knowing that God is working all these details into my life to make me better prepared for His work here and in heaven.

About noon, Ernestine checked my vitals. In our conversations, she told me about health concerns for which she was hesitant to see a doctor. I recounted how my annual check-up had led to early diagnosis of multiple myeloma before it invaded my body more extensively. We rejoiced with "Thank you, Jesus!" and Ernestine decided to get a check-up soon. Here I saw the fragrance of God's presence overpower the aroma of stem cell preservative.

Irma and Nancy arrived around 2 pm for a visit and to resupply me with clean clothes. I was wearing street clothes, not a hospital gown. Although I had not expected this, occasionally a staff member would come into my room and ask where the patient was; we would laugh when I identified myself. While Irma and I were alone, I was able to sneak a kiss, something that would not be allowed when I became neutropenic.

I learned about Irma's handling of things at home with some help from the family. Nancy told of experiences on their trip to Colorado, ranging from car sickness and detours to tent camping, dinners with friends, and surfing sand dunes. I described to Irma and Nancy how well I was feeling and how I was hopeful of God's continued grace as I faced the tougher days ahead. We decided to quarantine the main part of our home prior to my becoming an outpatient. On Wednesday, we would be instructed more fully about outpatient care.

Thus far in the stem cell transplant process, I was highly impressed by the medical staff associated with the SLU Blood and Marrow Transplant program. They knew what patients would experience along the way, explained this clearly to the patient, and took steps to either prevent or quickly manage problems. They monitored vital signs and blood status as my body traveled the recovery trajectory. They checked that I was diligent in exercise, drinking, eating, and watching for symptoms to help them do their work well. I knew that God determined the outcomes, but I also appreciated the expert care of these professionals.

Sunday, August 19, 2018 (Transplant Day +2)

I got up to be weighed and made myself a peanut butter and cracker snack before breakfast arrived. I took a 10-minute walk and 10-minute bike ride and then completed my assigned stretching exercises. I found encouragement from my Bible reading declaring how secure I am in my relationship with Jesus Christ. I was able to watch a videostream of the church service that I would normally attend. I sang along and learned about the dangers of a tongue that is out of control. I heard in the benediction reassuring words I had previously posted on my hospital room wall (Romans 15:13, NIV):

May the God of hope fill you with all joy and peace as you trust in him, so that you may overflow with hope by the power of the Holy Spirit.

Laura and Dr. Rajeh told me that my body was responding to the transplant as expected. Absolute neutrophils (baby stem cells) were dropping on their way to zero, but I was not yet neutropenic. Laura prescribed saline solution in anticipation of dehydrating side effects. Dr. Rajeh suggested that I might be more comfortable wearing pajamas than street clothes: "You look like you're preparing to leave." I assured him that I needed their expert care and planned to stay through this process.

Sunday afternoon I grabbed a book I had packed: *Stepping Up: A Call to Courageous Manhood*, by Dennis Rainey. I flipped to a chapter titled: "Are You Done Making a Difference?" A quote from Howard Hendricks caught my attention: "When your memories are more exciting than your dreams, you've begun to die." I read that older men should be active in families, communities, and life. Yes, I am responsible to God to use days He gives me to accomplish His purposes and prepare younger generations to do likewise. I wanted to use my journey with multiple myeloma to fulfill dreams and make a difference.

Mid-afternoon I called Irma to talk about the day's activities. She was being encouraged and helped by our friends at church. She missed a swim because no one joined her. My absence was missed.

Jeff and Jeanette from church stopped for a short visit with me. We had a wonderful time sharing things happening in our personal lives and families. I explained how my unexpected multiple myeloma diagnosis was such a blessing because it came before skeletal damage had occurred. We were reminded that God has been so very gracious in caring for each of us.

After a nice supper, I called my old friend Jack in Moscow, Idaho to bless him. His wife had passed away in March, so he lived alone on his wheat ranch. We enjoyed a short conversation about our families, gardens, and church. I explained my health situation beyond what he had heard through his church. I also thanked Jack for inspiring me in gardening and described a few of my gardening struggles. Jack responded by offering to send me special corn seed that he uses. I could see that Jack was supported by his children and their spouses, who were at that moment cooking corn from his garden for their evening dinner together.

I ended the day with a call to Irma for a final wrap-up and time in God's word.

Monday, August 20, 2018 (Transplant Day +3)

Overnight test results and observations showed no problems except some swelling in my feet. I took 5 pills this morning (antibacterial, antifungal, antiviral, stomach acid, etc.) I also received a 1000 mL saline solution drip.

Dan said Melphalan had a delayed killing effect on cells like Round-up® has on plants. Thus, I would be exhausted in 1-2 days, and neutropenic 1-2 days later. He said I would receive an injection probably on Transplant Day +5 to stimulate new neutrophil cell production to counter the worst losses.

Today Dr. Rajeh had a large team—nurse practitioners, doctor-in-training, RN, and pharmacist—just observing. After a few questions and looking into my mouth for sores, Dr. Rajeh said all was progressing well and he was hopeful that my recovery would go quickly. When he asked if they could do anything for me, I responded that we can be praying that God will bring me a speedy recovery. Dr. Rajeh ended with, "I am."

Irma visited in the afternoon. She brought me changes of clothes and updated me on the large harvest of beans from my garden. I missed being able to help harvest and do yard work. We discussed how my contributions at home and my interactions with the family would be limited for some time, which was a bit discouraging.

I was visited by the nursing team leader whom I had not met previously. When she asked me how I got here, I told her about my diagnosis, surgery, chemo, and stem cell transplant. I told her of kind and competent care that I had been receiving from nurses and other hospital workers. I acknowledged God's goodness in my early diagnosis, responses to treatments so far, and the vast number of people praying and supporting me in this venture.

I ended the afternoon with a ride on the stationary bike, going 2.3 virtual miles in 10 minutes at load incline level 2. It was a good way to unwind and remind myself that I still had energy to be active.

This was only Transplant Day +3 and I was beginning to tire of the long time being out of commission. And the worst was yet to come. As I waited for dinner, I remembered song sheets I had collected from our church's Sunday services and started to thumb through them. Words of the song, *Everlasting God*, spoke about **waiting** upon the Lord to gain His strength. I listened to a YouTube rendition of the song and noted comforting reassurances for those who wait upon the Lord:

> Strength will rise as we wait upon the Lord.
> Our God reigns forever: He is our hope, our strong deliverer.
> He is the everlasting God who does not faint or grow weary.
> He defends the weak and comforts those in need.
> He lifts us up on wings like eagles.

In my evening phone call with Irma, we both were feeling the disruptions in our lives. We found encouragement from the *Everlasting Father* song and from our reading from Genesis 45. Joseph who had been sold into slavery by his brothers years before stated to them, "It is not you who sent me here but God." Joseph was now in a position to save his relatives from starvation. We must remember that God puts us in places that may be uncomfortable at the time so that we might accomplish much greater things later. Irma and I must trust God in our current challenges.

I had been experiencing difficulty sleeping with nighttime interruptions and slowness going to sleep. I followed advice to use a sleep aid so I would be rested before I hit neutropenia and I would be interrupted more frequently.

Tuesday, August 21, 2018 (Transplant Day +4)

I wondered if my blood cell counts had taken their anticipated dive. I was a bit eager to reach the low point so I could begin recovery. Dan told me that counts had not changed much. Dr. Rajeh told me he found no concerns and that tomorrow I would receive an injection of Granix, a growth factor to mature white blood cells faster.

I felt that I must be proactive to prevent discouragement. I read in my Bible about God's promise to forgive sins and be our God. After breakfast I walked 10 minutes, did 10 stretching exercises, and took a 10-minute bike ride. I enjoyed music and Bible teaching on Christian radio. Due to some poor menu choices, I ate only part of my lunch.

Early afternoon, Tom the chaplain and I enjoyed posted Bible verses and relating them to needs of patients. I told Tom about God's kindness in my early cancer diagnosis and treatments. I shared insights I gained through the song and Bible reading from yesterday. He asked how Irma was doing. Tom was appreciative when I told him that I had prayed for him and other hospital chaplains this morning. We parted with commitments to trust God in our challenges ahead.

When Dan returned in mid-afternoon, I quizzed him about expectations as my blood counts dropped. He reminded me that each patient responds differently. I would experience fatigue, the extent of which may depend upon any gastrointestinal problems. He encouraged me to stay active even when I didn't feel strong.

I chatted with Irma in late afternoon before she got together with family for dinner. After dinner, we chatted again to update me on family activities and plan for Irma's visit the next day. We read (Genesis 45) about Joseph inviting his father's family to Egypt so they could survive five more years of famine. When his father Jacob realized that Joseph was alive, this lifted a huge burden so he could live his last years in peace. I thought "How small is my multiple myeloma load," and it too will end.

Approaching a low point in my blood counts, I reviewed their changes over pre-transplant chemo, transplant, and post-transplant periods. As shown, my counts were relatively stable during this time, apart from white cell and neutrophil absolute (ANC) peaks after the transplant. Days +1 through +4 white cells and neutrophils remained strong and stable, so infection was not a problem. Red cells (hemoglobin and hematocrit) were low but steady, not requiring a transfusion. Platelets were beginning to dip below normal, suggesting that I may need a platelet transfusion in the future.

I had weathered a week since Transplant Day -2 without suffering any

BLOOD COUNT TRENDS SINCE TRANSPLANT					
Test	Normal	Day 0	Day +1	Day +2	Day +4
White cells	3.5-10.5	8.7	10.5	6.4	5.5
Hemoglobin	13.5-17.5	10.6 (L)	10.1 (L)	10.2 (L)	10.1 (L)
Hematocrit	42.0-52	32.7 (L)	31.1 (L)	30.3 (L)	31.4 (L)
Platelets	150-400	174	170	155	140 (L)
ANC	1.6-7.0	8.3	10.1	6.2	5.2

serious problems. For this I was truly thankful.

Transplant Valley
Holding on for Life

I was approaching the point when my blood would be unable to support me adequately. Dangerous conditions that might require targeted responses were:

1. Neutropenia – Very low absolute neutrophil count and few white blood cells to fight infection leave the patient dangerously vulnerable. Neutrophil absolute count below 1.0×10^3 (1,000) may require white cell transfusion.
2. Thrombocytopenic – Very low blood platelet count makes the patient susceptible to dangerous bleeding. Platelets below 10×10^3 (10,000) require a platelet transfusion.
3. Anemia – Red blood cell count is too low so it limits oxygen transport to all parts of the body. Normal hemoglobin (Hgb) for men is between 14 and 18. Blood transfusion is required if hemoglobin falls below 8.

Wednesday, August 22, 2018 (Transplant Day +5)

My nurse practitioner Rachel informed me that my counts were beginning to fall, but I was not yet neutropenic. She said a delay before neutropenia was good in that it gave stem cells more time to produce new cells, and this might shorten the neutropenic period. Today I would receive IV fluids and an injection to stimulate white cell production.

Later Dr. Rajeh confirmed that I should reach neutropenia in a day or two. Since most neutropenic patients experience infections, we would need to be vigilant. I would receive IV fluids today to offset the high activity of my kidneys; I might be receiving IV fluids for several days. I might be ready to leave the hospital by the end of next week.

Irma and Nancy came for a meeting with Kim, the BMT discharge coordinator. From Kim it became clear that transplant recovery extends weeks beyond the inpatient portion, and patient and caregiver responsibilities are substantial.
- Patient is driven to BMT clinic for regular check-ups.
- Patient's fluid intake and output are recorded daily.
- We must alert BMT staff to signs of infections or illnesses.
- Sanitation at all times is paramount to avoid infections.
- Patient is driven to BMT when problems are suspected.

This was a reminder that we needed God's help in protecting me and in supporting my needs for weeks after discharge.

Nancy left for an interview, so Irma and I had time together, but not alone. I received a liter of saline solution for hydration and an injection of Granix to stimulate white cell growth. The dressing around my central line was replaced. I snacked on a protein drink. Irma and I took a "power" walk up and down the hallway. We reminded one another that our strength will rise as we wait upon the Lord. When Nancy returned, they went home.

My appetite was poor at suppertime, so I nibbled at a veggie burger and ate fruit. The day ended with my nighttime pills and an injection to prevent an upset stomach. I was in bed by 9 pm, hoping for a good night's sleep before I hit neutropenia. My bones felt "on edge" (probably from Granix) and kept me from sleeping, so I was given Ambien to treat insomnia, and later given Ativan to calm anxiety and help me sleep. I slept, but not as much as I had hoped.

Thursday, August 23, 2018 (Transplant Day +6)

When my white cell counts fell below 1 and ANC values fell below 1.0 ($x10^3$), I was neutropenic. A sign was placed outside my door (see photo). It felt hard to get out of bed, but that probably stemmed from lack of sleep. After I was up, my energy level felt normal. I was pleased to show the therapist consistent data on exercises, walking, and bike riding I had done each day.

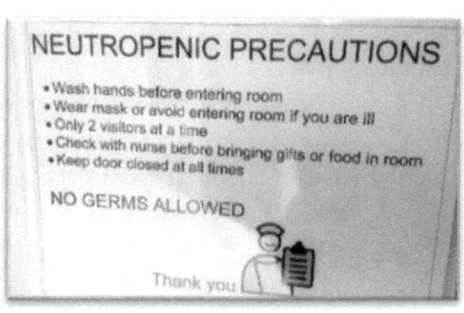

I received a liter of IV fluids to keep my hydration high. Dr. Rajeh said I would probably see lower blood counts for a day or two before they began increasing. The staff would take steps to control bone pain and enhance sleeping while I continued receiving Granix for a few more days. They would watch closely for signs of infection.

My appetite was relatively good today. Surprisingly, I ate most of my breakfast and lunch. I did not feel "wiped out" or discouraged.

Today I put on my wall an excerpt from Psalm 23, which talks of Jesus as our personal shepherd who cares for us (Psalm 23:4, NIV):

> "Even though I walk through the darkest valley, I will fear no evil for You are with me."

Indeed, my Good Shepherd was helping me through this dark valley.

I remained active within my neutropenic constraints. In my first walk, I wore a mask and was accompanied by my IV pole with the saline pouch doing its thing. After I had finished my IV drip and lunch, I had freedom to go for another walk, again wearing a medical mask (see selfie). I took a 10-minute ride on the stationary bike and traveled 2.1 virtual miles. Although I was getting exercise, I was also missing the walks and bike rides with Irma back home.

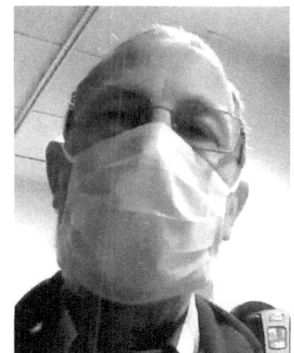

But God gave me a special treat! In mid-afternoon I received an email from my 12-year-old granddaughter Gloria to cheer me up. She told me about several of her activities, exuding with passion for doing challenging things in writing, music, and robotics. Her writing skill was obvious from the clarity and structure of her message. Her concern for me and my needs was also evident. This was the first email of encouragement I received from my grandkids, so it meant a lot to me.

Toward evening, I heard that most people experience infections that need immediate attention after inpatient care ends. In outpatient emergencies, we need to get to BMT within 30 minutes of reporting a problem and being told to come. This prompted my thoughts about inpatient/outpatient options:

1. Remain inpatient until I am able to drive, avoiding the need of drivers for emergency trips to SLU
2. Go outpatient and operate from home, having family transportation ready on a moment's notice.
3. Go outpatient and operate from home, depending on ambulance for emergency transport to SLU
4. Go outpatient and operate from a location near SLU until risks of infection are minimal, then go home and respond to emergencies if they occur.

Friday, August 24, 2018 (Transplant Day +7)

On Transplant Day +7, I saw signs that I was very near the bottom of the dark valley. Through the night, I experienced bone pain that kept me from sleeping until I received Ambien for sleep and oxycodone for pain. I felt moderate pain overall, but especially in hips and lower back. This told me that Granix was stimulating white cell production in my bones.

After being awakened by a 7 am thunder clap, I delayed getting up until 7:30 because I felt tired. Once I was up, got dressed, and had a snack, I felt normal again. Thank you, Lord, your mercies are new every morning.

Dan told me that my marker counts were nearly bottomed out: white cell counts were 0.1, and ANC was 60. My resistance to infection was essentially nil, so I must be extremely careful to avoid infections.

Dr. Rajeh indicated that this might be my lowest white cell counts; white cells should start increasing in a day or two. When I described my bone pain, he explained that Granix stimulates white cell growth. Because the hip region has the greatest bone concentration, it would be most affected by pain. He offered an additional pain reliever that could be taken tonight. My red blood counts and platelets were more slowly affected by chemo so they had not yet dropped significantly. Hopefully this meant I might avoid needing blood transfusions.

Dr. Rajeh was pleased with my progress and expected to see acceptable blood counts in a few days. To my surprise, he suggested next Tuesday (Day +11) for discharge from inpatient care. I expressed mixed feelings about that possibility: excited that I might be home soon but concerned about logistics. I explained that we would likely have difficulty getting to the BMT clinic within 45 minutes if an emergency occurred. He said we could delay discharge a few days until emergencies would be less probable.

My daily exercise was a bit different because I was told to wear a medical mask when outside of my room. I also had a saline solution drip that gave me a pole to drag along during part of my day. I did, however, complete my stretching exercises while the therapist watched, I took walks, and I rode the exercise bike. At one point, the nurse supervisor indicated that I should limit my walks to a hallway behind the nurses' station where the air was highly filtered and foot traffic was restricted.

Irma got a ride from Diane and Sandy at church to come after lunch for a short visit and resupply. She exchanged laundered for soiled clothes and brought me goodies: banana-chocolate-chip muffin, grapes, and grape juice. As we considered how I had felt well and had a good appetite during my journey into the valley, we thanked God for sustaining me beyond what we had expected.

Since I had eaten large meals at breakfast and lunch and a snack of grapes in the afternoon, I chose to snack for supper. I enjoyed my banana muffin, trail mix, string cheese, banana, and grape juice. It was nice having some fresh items not taken from the hospital menu.

In the evening I called Irma for our Bible reading from Genesis 47. Seeing that Jacob was 130 years old when his family moved to Egypt reminded me that God numbers our days and provides strength for those days. We could rest knowing that the One who created us could also sustain us. This was more relevant when I remembered that a man was shot and killed not far from the hospital that morning.

Saturday, August 25, 2018 (Transplant Day +8)

Throughout the night, my sleep was interrupted by discomfort in my bones. Although I took Ambien, oxycodone, and Ativan at different points in the night, the pain continued whenever I was in bed. When I got up, dressed, and became active in the morning, the pain disappeared and I could resume my regular activities. After exercise, breakfast, and visits from staff, I stole a morning nap to get rid of drowsiness.

In his rounds, Dr. Rajeh focused mostly on my blood counts and sleep issues. As shown, my neutrophil absolute had reached zero, while white cells, red cells, and platelets were all below normal. A transfusion might be required if red cells or platelets fell too much. Low cell counts had not affected my appetite or ability to exercise, but they made me much more conscientious about sanitation. Dr. Rajeh indicated that my counts should begin rising in a day or two.

BLOOD COUNTS SLIDING TO BOTTOM					
Test	Day +4	Day +5	Day +6	Day +7	Day +8
White cells	5.5	2.5 (L)	0.8 (L)	0.1 (L)	0.1 (L)
Hemoglobin	10.1 (L)	9.9 (L)	10.2 (L)	9.3 (L)	9.5 (L)
Hematocrit	31.4 (L)	29.0 (L)	30.7 (L)	29.6 (L)	28.5 (L)
Platelets	140 (L)	115 (L)	117 (L)	93 (L)	43 (L)
ANC	5.2	2.3	0.72 (L)	0.06 (L)	0 (L)

Dr. Rajeh was determined to help me sleep better so I could get rest I needed in my weakened condition. He made available another pain medication for use if I should be unable to sleep. It would be nice to be able to sleep without the distracting pain.

Even in a day with my cell counts bottomed out, I felt quite energetic and in good health. I walked at the normal pace, biked as I had been doing, and ate most of the food brought me.

I was encouraged by a phone call with Irma keeping one another updated. When I heard that she harvested two colanders of green beans, I felt a bit guilty for planting so many beans that she now had to harvest and preserve. Pastor Steve called to check on me, and we enjoyed recounting the many ways God had blessed me on this journey: minimal side effects, no infections, good energy and appetite, and opportunities to share God's goodness with others.

Sunday, August 26, 2018 (Transplant Day +9)

Transplant Day +9 started rough due to lack of sleep. Before going to bed, the medical staff planned to continue my pills for sleeping and bone pain, but add an injection when sleep alluded me. Around 11 pm, I called for the injection and waited to see how it worked: It did not work. Two hours later, I decided against another injection. From that time until 4 am, my temperature and blood pressure rose a bit and I slept little. Around 4 am my body began to relax and I slept more. By 7:30 am I was up, dressed, ate a banana and snack bar, and was feeling more normal again. But I could tell that if I sat quietly in my chair with my eyes closed, I would soon doze off.

When breakfast arrived, it was not what had ordered, but I enjoyed the small quiche and orange juice and milk. I got a text from Irma stating that she was exhausted from lack of sleep. I advised her to stay home from church and both of us could watch the videostream of the service from our respective locations. At first the audio from the church was not working. When the audio began working, we heard most of Pastor Steve's message about using the tongue to bless others. Lord, how can I bless Irma when I am weakened and in the hospital?

Dr. Rajeh and Megan were baffled about my sleeping problems, saying that I needed to identify the causes (pain, anxiety, etc.) so meds could be prescribed to address the correct problem. My white cell and ANC counts remained at zero. Red cells and platelets had not fallen enough to require transfusions.

I took a nap and completed my stretching exercises before a nice lunch of chowder and beef stroganoff. Bible teaching and music on BBN radio helped me remember God's faithfulness through my treatment journey. In the afternoon, I napped and rode the exercise bike 2.25 miles at level 2. I was pleased that my energy was holding up.

When I called Irma, she appeared more rested. As we talked about the next few days, we realized that transition to outpatient status this week might require us to find alternatives to her driving me to appointments at SLU. I encouraged her to talk to the family to see what options we may have. Knut might have the family car for a week, during which time our car would be called upon to meet a variety of transportation needs.

Megan came to discuss a plan for addressing my sleep problem. Dr. Rajeh approved a combination of Ambien and an IV injection of Dilaudid (hydromorphone hydrochloride), an opioid narcotic pain reliever, to remove distracting pain. The hope was to get me asleep early and then quickly to sleep after awakening. Megan was committed to giving me a good night's sleep; she stated that if the meds don't work, she would 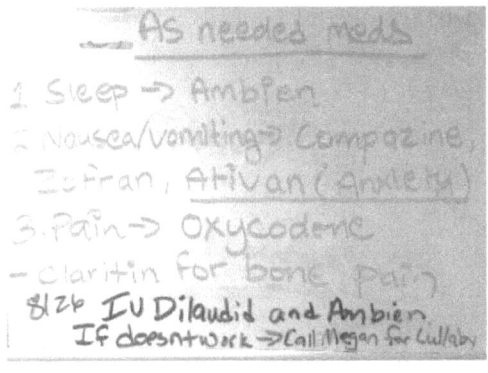 sing me a lullaby (see bottom of whiteboard photo). I appreciated the efforts of the staff, but also knew that in the end the Lord determines how my night would go.

Monday, August 27, 2018 (Transplant Day +10)

Transplant Day +10 got off to a great start. Megan was spared a call for a lullaby! The narcotic injection calmed my aching (and at times, jabbing) pain in my flesh so that I slept peacefully for about 2 hours before the effect wore off and the cycle repeated. Even with interruptions every 2 hours, I felt that I was resting and being refreshed.

Bennie took the midnight blood sample. At my 4:30 am injection, she reported that my platelets count was 7 (see table), below the required 10, so I needed a transfusion. She promptly ordered a unit of platelets and gave me a half-hour transfusion. A post-transfusion blood sample showed my platelets count rose to 20, so all was well again.

8/27/2018 BLOOD CELL COUNT		
Test	Normal	Mine
White cells	3.5-10.5	0.1 (L)
Hemoglobin	13.5-17.5	9.1 (L)
Hematocrit	42.0-52.0	26.9 (L)
Platelets	150-400	7 (LL)
Neutrophil Abs	1.6-7.0	0.03 (LL)

When morning arrived, Dan told me that although white cells did not increase, ANC rose from 0 the previous day to 30. (Perhaps engrafting had begun). Because stem cells have begun to produce neutrophils, white cell count should increase soon. Although I was encouraged, I was cautioned that my susceptibility to infections was very high while my white cell counts were essentially zero. The battle was not over, but the stem cell troops were beginning to engage in the battle.

Dr. Rajeh and Dan stopped by late morning. As I told them my experience with the latest pain medication, I began to realize that I had had the same type of pain, but lower level, after receiving Neupogen injections prior to apheresis. Stimulated stem cell activity in my bones had produced bone and body pain. Dr. Rajeh told me the current state of my bone marrow likely resulted in greater pain than when marrow was healthy. He said we would stop Granix injections as soon as my white counts were acceptable.

I asked Dr. Rajeh what I might expect now that my ANC was starting to rise. He responded that it would take a few days for my white counts to reach an acceptable level; I might be ready for discharge toward the end of the week. He also expected my platelets to drop again so that I might need another platelet transfusion.

After lunch, Pastor Steve came to visit. Wearing a medical mask didn't slow his questions on topics including how Irma and I were doing, what I was learning through my cancer experience, and what were the essentials of the gospel. He stated that many "Christians" do not grasp that people are separated from God and unable to bridge this gap on our own; we all needed supernatural intervention of God through Jesus Christ to open the way. We discussed my intent to publish a book on my cancer experience and my desire to finish life well prepared for heaven. I appreciated his offers of help and his prayer.

I had a brief nap, then a visit from Chaplain Tom. After I updated him on my health, we discussed issues that would arise when I became an outpatient. He suggested that we talk with the social worker to see if housing and transportation options in the area might help us through the most stressful times.

Nancy brought Irma to the hospital, then went to attend a music workshop in the area. Today's visit from 4:30 to 8 pm gave Irma and me time to discuss things more deeply than in previous days. It was also good to have face-to-face time together reading from the Bible and praying.

With discharge possible later in the week, Irma and I discussed options for transition to outpatient status. Dan indicated that I might be able to drive immediately after inpatient discharge. If I were allowed to drive, we could easily accommodate outpatient visits with uncertain end times. Thank you, Lord, for solving our transportation problem.

As evening arrived, I found myself wanting to be very careful not to get sick, which might delay my discharge or increase my medication load due to an infection. When my nose required blowing, I remembered a support person who sniffled in my room that morning, saying it was just allergies. I noticed that my temperature reached 99F, when my normal was usually less than 98F. About 10 pm I experienced a 30-second shivering spell. Later I realized that in these fear-driven moments, I was not trusting the Lord. We were to tell the Lord our cares, with thanksgiving, and trust Him to resolve any fears in His way and time.

Tuesday, August 28, 2018 (Transplant Day +11)

Tuesday I started the day a bit tired. I had not consistently called for meds throughout the night, so I awoke more frequently and waited longer than I should to get my pain injection. After dressing and consuming a snack bar, I was hooked to a potassium supplement for 4 hours. Starting the infusion at 7 am, I missed taking a walk before breakfast.

Dan reported that my white cell count rose from 0.1 the day before to 0.3. My absolute neutrophil count rose from 30 to 190, beginning a significant upward trend. My potassium level had fallen to 3.4, below the limit of 3.5, which required the potassium supplement.

Dr. Rajeh came around noon to discuss my progress and next steps. He confirmed that I would be allowed to drive (if a caregiver was with me) after he had released me. My discharge date might be this week or next, depending on my health status. If I were transfusion-dependent (facing a possible blood or platelet transfusion) at discharge, I would be required to stay locally to minimize travel time and stress of getting to BMT outpatient services. Once I became transfusion-independent, I would be allowed to drive to outpatient services from home.

This new information led to discussions with Irma about merits of the two options and possible nearby lodging. Irma and I both wanted to get me out of the hospital as soon as it was safe. We felt we could stay nearby and live out of a suitcase for a few days if I drove and we had places to walk and things to do nearby. At this point Irma and I were leaning toward the discharge while transfusion-dependent option.

I did my regular exercises at levels comparable to earlier days. However, I found myself wondering if exercises were more tiring than previously. Looking at my blood counts, I saw that hemoglobin dropped from 10.2 to 8.9 in the last 5 days, a 13 percent drop. If it dropped to 8.0, I would need a transfusion. I recalled that Dr. Rajeh said a transfusion for platelets was yet likely. My hemoglobin and platelets counts would determine when I became transfusion-independent.

I looked online for motels where we might stay on the weekend if I was discharged at the end of the week. Many motels were not available on these dates. I learned that the St Louis Cardinals were playing home games Friday, Saturday, and Sunday, so lodging would be difficult to find.

By the end of the day, I changed my preference to discharge when transfusion-independent. With this option, Irma and I could avoid needs for finding local lodging, finding ways to feed ourselves, and getting our car to the hospital to use locally. Yes, a transfusion-independent discharge would suit us best.

Wednesday, August 29, 2018 (Transplant Day +12)

Transplant Day +12 got off to a good start. My night nurse Cait told me that my blood cell counts looked good, so I was hopeful that my discharge would be sooner rather than later. I noticed bruises and blemishes on my hands (due to low platelets) and wondered what other side effects I might yet experience. When I saw the occasional hair on the table in front of me, I wondered if I would yet see significant hair loss. I needed to remind myself that God was in control and He knew me even down to the number of hairs on my head.

I got up feeling relatively rested, even though I had awakened about every hour and requested pain meds every 2 hours. I ate a snack bar and graham crackers with peanut butter when I got up. I also ate a big breakfast of English muffin, sausage patty, orange juice, raisin bran, and milk. Yes, my appetite was good.

Dan reported that my white cell count had risen from 0.3 to 0.9, showing encouraging progress. Hemoglobin stayed at 8.9 rather than continuing to drop, perhaps suggesting that we could avoid a transfusion required at 8.0. Platelets dropped from 15 to 12, a much smaller drop than the previous day; this indicated that platelet production had kicked in, so another transfusion might be avoided.

My ANC jumped from .19 to .73, now above .50 so I was no longer severely neutropenic, just neutropenic. If tomorrow's increase was the same, I would no longer be neutropenic and might soon be eligible for discharge. In the meantime, Granix injections would cease.

Stephanie my daytime nurse commented that I seemed to have it pretty good. I was taking a small number of pills and experiencing few problems. Jokingly, I told her I was here on vacation. Seeing the Scripture verses posted on the wall, she asked if I was a Christian. I explained that my trust in Jesus Christ is my strength through this journey.

Dr. Rajeh, accompanied by several medical interns, summarized my status. My blood counts looked good: white cells were up, ANC was up, and platelets were showing signs of stabilizing. I might be transfusion-independent by Friday and be allowed to go home. Because my condition had changed so positively, Dr. Rajeh spoke of my going home rather than staying nearby for a few days. I thanked him for such good news, and he said he was pleased to be the messenger of good news. Indeed, I was encouraged.

Irma got a ride with Nancy from our church and came to replenish my wardrobe. Of course we were delighted with the likelihood that I might be home that week.

In the evening, I called Irma and we chatted about our expectations for my discharge. We had been told by many that recovery would take multiple months, but we were hoping for a much faster recovery. Our Bible reading (Genesis 49) reminded us that great heroes of the faith experienced hard times to prepare them for purposes of God. We wondered what our cancer experience might be preparing us to do. Knowing God's faithfulness and His love for His children, we could rejoice now anticipating that He was doing something good that we might not yet see.

Thursday, August 30, 2018 (Transplant Day +13)

When I called Gabrielle after midnight for pain meds, she provided help with my pain and then told me that my tests showed that I was no longer neutropenic. My platelets had also begun to increase, averting the need for a transfusion. I interpreted this to mean that I would be transfusion-independent, allowing me to be discharged tomorrow (Friday). I praised the Lord for these amazing results.

I was up at 6:30 am, tired but ready to get moving. Dan explained my test results. My ANC of 1.26 put me out of the neutropenic state and showed that neutrophils had increased over .50 two days in a row. Platelets increased from 12 to 16, reversing a downward trend and avoiding the need for a transfusion. White cells increased the third day in a row. Red cell counts remained unchanged. These conditions suggested that neither platelets nor red cells would require a transfusion—making me transfusion-independent so I could go home. Cell count increases the third day in a row indicated that stem cell engraftment had occurred on Transplant Day +10. Praise God for getting me to this state so quickly.

I asked Dan about the discharge process and its timing. He told me that hospital personnel would discharge me and send me home, possibly by 2 or 3 in the afternoon. I would receive additional instructions for follow-up appointments at the BMT outpatient clinic.

Dan cautioned me that at home I should attempt to mitigate risks. I could do what I felt capable of doing, but should not subject myself to potential infections, especially exotic ones. I would not need to wear a mask under most conditions, but should avoid environments that presented hazards from bacteria, fungi, and viruses. Dan cited an example of a post-transplant farmer who contracted a disease from his chickens and he died. My body would need time to develop immunities, including those that I had before my transplant.

Dr. Rajeh told me that, barring surprises in tonight's blood tests, I would be transfusion-independent and could be discharged tomorrow. I would return to the BMT outpatient clinic on Saturday or Sunday for a check-up. When I asked him what I might expect next, he responded with, "Hair loss". He said that each person is different, but hair loss could occur at this point in recovery. I would not need to wear a face mask, but I should be ready to wear one where infectious agents were likely present.

I called Irma to report what I had learned. She now was able to arrange transportation for my journey home.

I began to realize that the transplant recovery process and its dangers were not yet behind me. I found myself thinking about how different conditions or decisions would affect me and my ability to do things I wanted to do. I was still hoping to be able to travel, such as to attend the IRE Advisory Board meeting in Minnesota. I had to remind myself that I must trust God and seek His direction in decisions before me. The Lord watches over me, protects me, and enables me to do whatever He wants me to do.

Dan returned to tell me that he would be off duty on Friday so he would not be present when I was discharged. His replacement would walk me through the discharge process and schedule my appointment at the BMT clinic after Dr. Rajeh approved my discharge. When I asked Dan how my transplant process compared with others, he said my process was exceptionally smooth with few bumps, even considering the huge chemo dose I received. When I asked Dan about my travel restrictions, he indicated that if all went well, I should be able to drive to Minnesota in 3 weeks.

Finally, I thanked Dan for his excellent work and asked if I could pray for us. In my prayer, I praised God for Dan and his expert care, and I thanked God for sustaining and healing me to-date and in the treatments to come.

I rode the stationary bike at a pace that pushed me. At the end of 10 minutes at a load level of 2, I travelled 2.25 virtual miles, as many as any other 10-minute period I had ridden, and my energy was not overtaxed. This encouraged me that I might be able to return to biking at home.

I was very pleased with my ability to stay active during my transplant process. As shown below, each day as an inpatient I completed my physical therapy exercises at least once, walked 10-minutes usually twice, and rode 1.5 to 4 miles on the exercise bicycle.

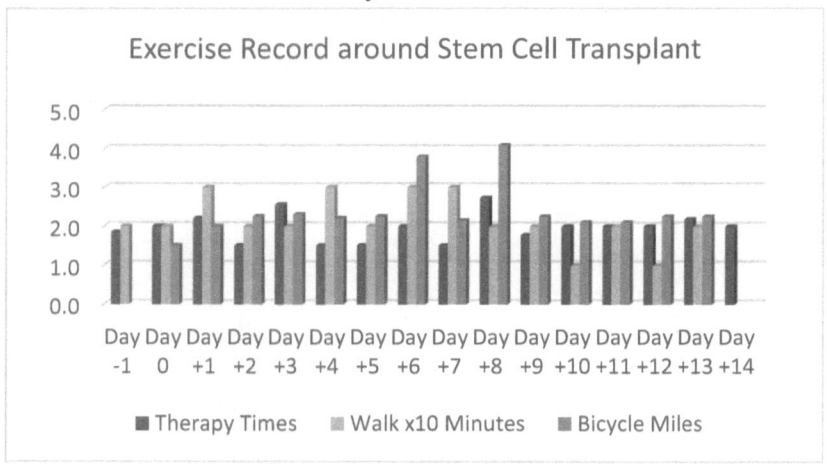

I called Irma after dinner. We shared our excitement about my going home the next day, but we also realized that our lives would be different. I needed time to regain energy and immunity to diseases. We would need to monitor my health and practice meticulous sanitation. We surely would face new challenges, but God would help us along the way.

Outpatient Recovery
Learning a New Normal

Going home was exciting but it also created new challenges. I would be around many people, including children of all ages. I would not be in highly sanitary conditions at all times. I might feel well, but I would need to be cautious about what I chose to do. I would not have expert medical care at my fingertips. I would have new opportunities, but also new responsibilities for minimizing risk of relapse or complications.

Friday, August 21, 2018 (Transplant Day +14)

Transplant Day +14 was my day of discharge from inpatient care at St Louis University Hospital.

Jessica, my nurse practitioner for the day, told me the steps and timing for the day. She said I might be discharged between noon and 2 pm. I called Irma to inform her of the hospital's plan so she and Nancy could finalize travel plans.

Shalu was my RN for my final day. She had been my nurse when I was admitted and a number of times in between. I expressed my appreciation for her wonderful care; indeed, she was possibly the one who served me most conscientiously during my stay. I took the opportunity to pray for her, thanking God for her care and skill and thanking Him for taking care of me. She responded that my prayer was very special to her.

Approval for my discharge was based on blood tests giving evidence that my health was stable enough for me to travel from home to the BMT clinic as needed. The table shows critical levels for hemoglobin, platelets, and neutrophil absolute. Although my counts were below the normal

8/31/2018 BLOOD CELL COUNT			
Test	Normal	Critical	Mine
White cells	3.5-10.5		2.3 (L)
Hemoglobin	13.5-17.5	>8.0	9.2 (L)
Hematocrit	42.0-52.0		27.2 (L)
Platelets	150-400	>10	18 (LL)
ANC	1.6-7.0	>1.0	1.17 (L)

ranges, they had increased above the critical levels to the point where transfusions of hemoglobin or platelets should not be required. This meant that I was transfusion-independent and could be discharged to go home.

When Dr. Rajeh made his rounds, he said I was going home. He told me the transplant process had gone smoothly with no infections, and I was a wonderful patient. I would need to drink lots of fluids, perhaps 3 liters per day, during recovery. I would see him next on Sunday in the BMT clinic (later this was changed to Saturday).

I thanked Dr. Rajeh and his team for their personal care and treatments to help me be successful. I asked him if I could pray for them, and with his approval I prayed. I thanked God for the expertise and care the team displayed for me and others in the unit, thanked God for protecting and strengthening me, and prayed for God's continued blessing on us. The team parted with smiles and expressions of appreciation for my prayer.

The discharge process included equipping me to be successful at home. I received a Walgreen's bag with blood pressure tester, thermometer, pill organizer box, sunscreen, face masks, and other care items. I received a revised pharmaceuticals list and script to obtain oxycodone from a pharmacy to control bone pain.

After lunch, Irma and Nancy arrived at the front of the hospital, where Shalu helped me get my stuff loaded into the car. Shalu gave me a goodbye hug, I hopped in the back seat, and Nancy drove Irma and me home.

Reaching home, Irma and I began the transition. We unpacked my stuff, organized pills for the remainder of the week, and set up a place for me to nap where I would not interfere with Irma's work. This also provided me a bed if I was restless at night and needed to leave our bed so as not to keep Irma awake. Irma and I went for a short walk, which made me realize how I had missed our walks together holding hands.

By dinner time, I began to see how emotional the day had been. I had said good-bye to many medical staff I had gotten to know and appreciate. I stepped out of the hospital into the world of sounds, smells, and sights that I had missed for two weeks. I once again enjoyed the dishes Irma prepared, with her special flair for taste and nutrition rolled into one. Each bite of familiar foods was so satisfying.

In the evening, I was surprised by a call from my brother Bob and his wife Jean. I had failed to email them of my discharge plans, so they assumed I had been home for a while. Because they and my brother Arnie and wife Judy were planning to visit us in October, the call was to start planning for this trip. It was clear that we needed to think more about activity Irma and I could handle in late October.

Saturday, September 1, 2018 (Transplant Day +15)

I had an appointment at the BMT outpatient clinic at 10 am on Saturday. I did not sleep well the night before, so I was very tired. Several times as I drove us to the clinic and back my alertness and responses to traffic conditions were not safe. I was surprised and shocked at how poorly I was driving. But God kept us safe and I assumed that my driving would be better once I had more sleep.

At the clinic, my blood tests showed that I was doing very well. In fact, Jamie told us that my next appointment would be Wednesday (4 days away), which delighted us! We had expected a checkup in one or two days. When our appointment ended, Irma and I ate our lunch in a patio seating area and we reflected on how well things were progressing. Dr. Rajeh walked by thinking that we had left before he had a chance to see me, so he stopped to chat when he saw us. He was pleased to see my continued improvements in test results.

Blood test results from the first day of high-dose chemotherapy to my

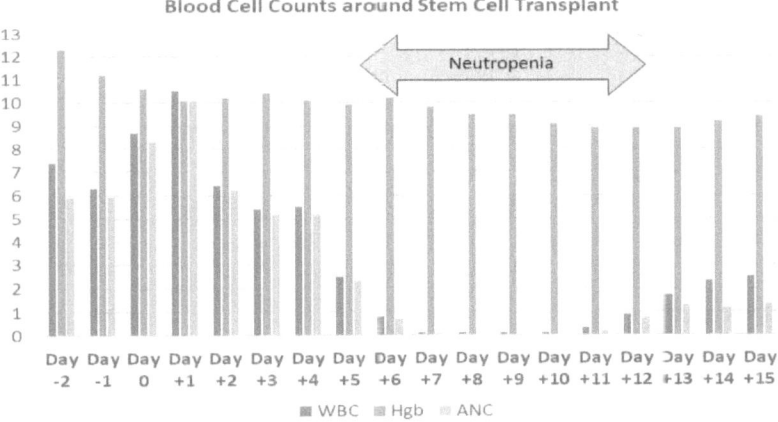

first outpatient checkup are graphed. These show how white cells and absolute neutrophil counts bottomed out and red cells dipped after the chemo kicked in. Neutropenia struck when ANC was below 1.0. My cell counts allowed me to go home, but they still needed time to return to normal levels.

Back home we felt our way into a new normal. My energy and alertness were diminished. I was giving more attention to following careful practices to avoid possible sources of infection. On an encouraging note, Irma and I were able to enjoy walks up to a mile at a good pace.

I continued to have bone pain. When I had been told much earlier about the possibilities of experiencing bone pain, I had no understanding of what that meant. I was now seeing that the achiness I experienced in earlier stages of the transplant process, which I thought was mostly stiff joints, was probably bone pain. My bone pain was an irritating ache from areas of my body that had boney structures, especially hips, legs, and lower back, with occasional jabs of pain and numbness in tissue around these areas or other parts of my body.

Irma helped me to see bone pain in a more positive sense. Pain was probably an indication that my stem cells were working overtime to rebuild my destroyed blood production system. Indeed, my cell counts were steadily climbing. Irma described this activity as the stem cells doing a celebration dance in my bones.

We saw from hair and beard shedding that significant hair loss had begun, and I was beginning to look shabby (as shown). Irma trimmed my beard to decrease its shagginess. At this point, we did not know how extensive hair loss would be, but we wanted to be ready for whatever occurred. I reminded myself that God knows the number of hairs on my head, and He controls what happens here.

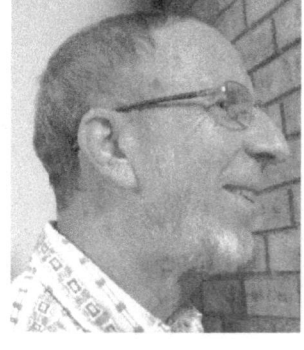

Sunday, September 2, 2018 (Transplant Day +16)

Sunday started off more traumatically than I expected. I had been awake and walked a lot during the night due to bone pain. In the morning while washing my hair, I felt a strange consistency in the shampoo and saw hair tangled with my fingers. Then I realized that I was losing a lot of hair here and now.

I piled tufts of hair outside the sink so it wouldn't clog the drain. I asked Irma to comb out the loose hair. My day's harvest was a sizable hairstack (see photo), or as Irma called it, a rat's nest. I kept the stack by the sink for the day so I could properly mourn my loss.

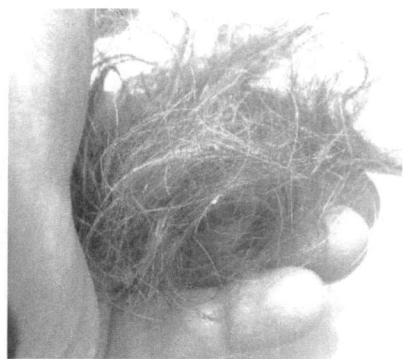

After a Sunday morning walk, Irma and I decided to stay home and watch the church service via livestream. We could sing with the congregation and hear the message without driving 25 minutes each way. We did not want my attendance to be a major distraction to our friends. Staying home also allowed morning and afternoon naps.

Irma and I began to verbalize questions regarding my recovery period. Would I isolate myself due to hair loss? I decided: No way! How long would hair loss last? How long would I need to wait before I had better sleeping and less bone pain? How much rest did I need? How much travel could I handle?

That day we received the anticipated email invitation to a Canadian Thanksgiving reunion of Irma's family near London, Ontario on October 6. I wanted to go, but as we discussed the uncertainty of my health, the 12-hour drive each way, crossing international borders, being on a farm with chickens and horses, and possibly needing out-of-country healthcare, we decided that taking this trip would be unreasonable. We regrettably declined, citing my health as our principal reason.

The late October visit from my brothers and their wives in conjunction with their trip to Branson, MO, was another travel question. We decided to be cautious, minimize our travel time, and yet maximize time with them. We would simply join them for a day or two in Branson, rather than having them drive between Mascoutah and Branson one-way or round trip.

Monday, September 3, 2018 (Transplant Day +17)

I had pain again Sunday night, but less than the previous night. I took one oxycodone pill at bedtime and none after that. With less pain, I walked and stretched less and slept more than the night before. After breakfast and a good walk, I felt good. I managed to have morning and afternoon naps.

For the second day Irma combed out my loose hair. The uneven tan on my head became more obvious so I began using our early morning walk to get a bit of sun on my head without risk of sunburn. I heard two different perspectives on my hair loss: Irma said it made me look older; Josh said it made me look younger. I thought it made me look balder. It definitely made my hats fit looser on my head.

After a long absence, I finally returned to some professional activities. I began working with Peter at OSU toward a journal article based on our Capstone Design Conference workshop. I also emailed my decision not to attend the Advisory Board meeting for the Iron Range Engineering program in northern Minnesota. In light of my health and limited activity in engineering education, I regretfully offered my resignation from this Advisory Board. This decision was emotional since I had been a part of this innovative program since before its inception 10 years earlier. It hurt to see multiple myeloma bringing a premature sunset to my professional involvements.

Bob and Jean called to firm up plans for their trip to Branson. We agreed that they and Arnie and Judy would travel directly to Branson on October 23. Irma and I would meet them there on October 25 and stay that night in Branson. That would allow them more time enjoying Branson, and we could restrict our participation to activities that fit our energy and interests.

Tuesday, September 4, 2018 (Transplant Day +18)

Tuesday began with new challenges. When we arose at 5:30 am, Irma said she was sick and may need to go to emergency. She explained that yesterday's pains in her shoulder and back had worsened and kept her from sleeping. Her mind was running wild about the problem: possible heart attack, cancer, etc.

Irma contacted an online doctor, and I texted Nancy to see if she could come over. The online doctor told Irma to see her primary care doctor. Nancy made sure my health was monitored while Irma was gone. In the end, Irma's doctor assured her that the pain was probably muscle related. She came home with steroid meds to help reduce the muscle pain. Thank you, Lord, for lifting the emotional load that had come on top of all my medical concerns.

The Robo Raiders met in our home, but I stayed away except for a short conversation in mask with three of the team's mentors. The 10-member team was planning how to best manage a 3-day high-intensity design-and-build session (robot in 3 days, or Ri3D) to start on Saturday. Their goal was to design and build a simple robot that performed key functions needed for this season's game. After having been a part of Ri3D activities in past years, I felt left out this year.

After supper, Irma and I went for a 2-3 mile bicycle ride out into the country and a loop through streets near home. This was my first ride after coming home, so I had wondered if I would be steady and had energy for riding. I shortened our ride as my energy began to drop, thinking that my low hemoglobin was limiting my energy.

Wednesday, September 5, 2018 (Transplant Day +19)

Wednesday was a very encouraging day. Irma slept through most of Tuesday night, not experiencing the pain that troubled her the night before. I slept quite well from 9 pm to midnight, and better after midnight than the night before. I was glad that I was not sleep-deprived since I would be driving to SLU that morning.

Before breakfast Irma brushed my head to remove loose hair so I would not shed in the house. My head was now nearly bald on top. The darker hair had fallen out, so only fine hair light in color remained. My appearance was clearly changing.

After a quick morning nap, I drove to the BMT outpatient clinic and back home without any problems. My appointment at the clinic was for replacing the dressing over my central line, checking my blood cell counts, and providing any treatments needed. As we waited for test results, Irma and I told Jamie about our outpatient practices. When we mentioned our bicycle ride, Jamie warned me to wear a helmet and avoid falling because my low platelets could cause me to bleed a lot.

I requested that I might be able to stop recording my intake and output, which I felt was unnecessary if I continued my disciplined water consumption. After Jamie studied my daily intake-output log, she relaxed this requirement.

When Jamie obtained my blood test results, she happily said they were "wonderful." Since Saturday, white cells increased from 2.5 to 6 and were now in the middle of the normal range. My ANC absolute had increased from 1.3 to 2.4, now well within the normal range. Red cell counts had increased about 7%, but remained below the normal range.

Irma and I were encouraged by Jamie's enthusiasm and by white cell counts, my ability to fight infections, in normal ranges. Jamie went on to say that I did not need to return for a checkup until Monday (5 days away) when we could also remove the central line. Wow! We were surprised by the difference between what we had expected (2-3 days to return) and the actions proposed by Jamie (5 days to return plus removal of central line). Jamie also said I could ride my bike without excessive concerns about bleeding. We were elated!

As Irma and I ate lunch in the Cancer Center patio, we praised God for His work in my body. It was not luck, diet, grit, and exercise that produced such good blood counts. God increased productivity of my engrafted stem cells and protected me from infections. We were moving toward a quick completion of the stem cell transplant process.

After returning home, Irma swam, then she and I added chlorine to shock the pool and moved solar covers in place to extend swimming a few days. After dinner we took a bicycle ride, bringing closure on an eventful and encouraging day.

Thursday, September 6, 2018 (Transplant Day +20)

Thursday began without my hoped-for "sleep through the night." I had experienced restless bones in the middle of the night, then ended with good sleep. In the morning I felt like doing garden work, but Irma warned me not to expose myself to bacteria, fungi, or viruses.

My brother Arnie and wife Judy called to get a firsthand report on my health and to assure us that we had a place to stay in Branson when we travelled there on October 25. Describing my unbelievably rapid stem cell engrafting and improved blood counts reminded me of God's goodness.

The Robo Raiders team met at our house to prepare for attending the FTC season kickoff in St Louis on Saturday. At the kickoff, they would have an opportunity to demonstrate robots, network with other teams, and see the field and rules for this year's robot game. Regrettably, I would remain home to stay away from crowds, but this meant I would also miss this launch of the robot season.

Friday, September 7, 2018 (Transplant Day +21)

Friday followed a good sleep with only short times awake during the night. I was beginning to accept my new appearance due to hair loss. Irma and I felt that my hair loss had stopped; remaining hair looked like fine reddish baby hair. The three photos show my hair changes over the last 6 months. We wondered how much hair would return, when, and what color and texture it would be.

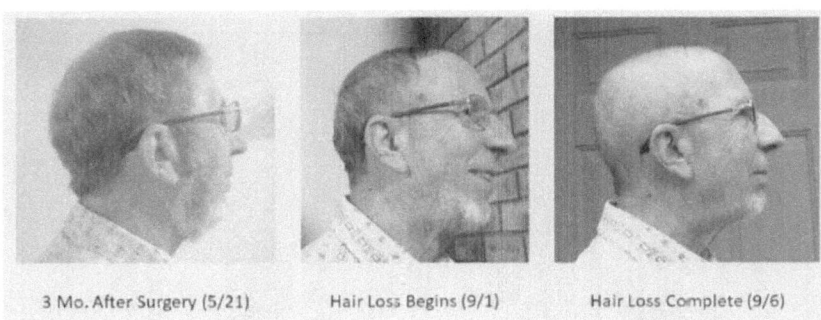

3 Mo. After Surgery (5/21)   Hair Loss Begins (9/1)   Hair Loss Complete (9/6)

Irma and Nancy and her two youngest kids swam while I cautiously hoed a few weeds in the strawberries and skimmed leaves from the pool. Later Irma and I vacuumed the pool and covered it with solar covers to hold heat for possible future swims. After supper, Irma and I took a bike ride into the country to get some fresh air and exercise.

To my surprise, I received a lovely "get well" card from the Missouri FTC Committee, which plans and oversees all of Missouri's FTC competitions. Because I had previously volunteered and coached our team at Missouri competitions, I knew many of the people who signed the card. I was touched by their thoughtfulness.

Saturday, September 8, 2018 (Transplant Day +22)

Saturday I stayed home while the Robo Raiders reportedly represented us very well at the FTC kickoff in St Louis. After the season's game was revealed, the Robo Raiders returned to our home to strategize and begin designing robots for the season. I wore my medical mask as I interacted with team members and coaches through the afternoon and evening. It felt good to contribute in a small way to get the team started on this year's robot design journey.

Knut was home from college for the weekend. Just for fun, he and Joe, both alumni of the Robo Raiders, designed and built their own robot for the FTC game. They labored to have a working robot before the weekend ended and Knut and Joe had to return to college.

As my transplant recovery period continued, I prepared a timeline (shown) to display the timing of major events associated with my stem cell transplant. One month had elapsed since my stem cell collection (aphere-

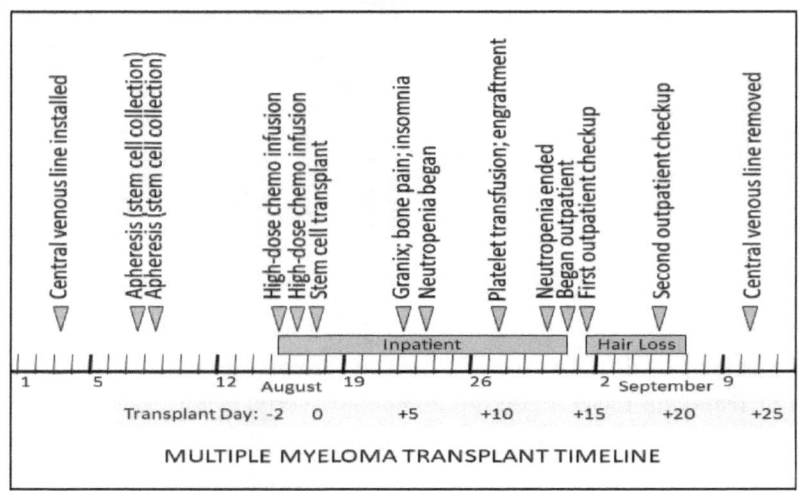

sis). Stem cell engraftment occurred 10 days after transplant. Two weeks of that time were spent as an inpatient watching my blood cell counts drop after chemo and then begin to rebound. My time at home had been interrupted by surprises related to hair loss and bone pain, but I had no infections. My central venous catheter had been in place for just over a month.

Sunday, September 9, 2018 (Transplant Day +23)

Sunday started after moderately good sleep for me but perhaps less for Irma. Since I had not attended church the past three Sundays, we really wanted to attend this day. My wearing a mask and sporting a peach fuzz hairdo made it difficult to slip in unnoticed. What joy it was to receive smiles, hugs, handshakes, and blessings of friends who had been praying for us for weeks. We had the opportunity to tell many about the goodness of God in seeing me through weeks of transplant and recovery. Singing while wearing a mask was difficult, but all the same, praise for God needed to come out in songs of worship.

Conversations with friends and acquaintances enabled us to encourage one another. When Jane introduced herself to me as a cancer survivor who understood what I was experiencing, I suddenly realized that I was now a "cancer survivor." I was one who had experienced cancer and its devastating impacts, and had a story to tell. I saw that people going through cancer treatments needed cancer survivors to assure them that they too could survive and live a fairly normal life.

Irma spent time talking to Peggy, another cancer survivor. Her robust health was encouraging, even after she told of some very difficult treatment experiences. We learned that my peach fuzz hair was quite common after people lose their hair; it would be months before new hair began to grow. I was beginning to accept my new hairdo.

After dinner, Irma and I enjoyed watching Knut and Joe show off their "robot in 30 hours." Although clearly a work-in-progress, their robot could collect game elements and score them, as well as hang itself at the end of the game. They posted videos of their robot in action on YouTube; we heard later that their videos had received thousands of views in a few days.

As Irma and I prepared waffles for supper, Nancy popped in before she took Knut back to college. She had skimmed my multiple myeloma story (draft of this book) which I had sent her the previous night. I was pleased to hear that my story was finding a place in her teaching her children from the book of James in the Bible: "Consider it pure joy when you encounter various trials . . . ." My story was enhancing their study of Scripture! Praise God!

Monday, September 10, 2018 (Transplant Day +24)

Monday followed moderately good sleep: up 3-4 times in the night, and I stayed in bed without bone restlessness. I drove us to the BMT clinic for a checkup and removal of my central line catheter. After seeing my blood test results, Laura described my progress as "fabulous." White cell counts were in the normal range and steady. I had none of the side effects she asked about: nausea, vomiting, poor appetite, diarrhea, constipation, fevers, headaches, rashes, mouth sores, etc. My reduced energy was what I had been told would happen. I assumed that my energy was going to replenishing cells in my body destroyed by chemotherapy.

Due to my fabulous recovery, I did not need additional treatment this day. Laura told me that in a week I would meet with her and Dr. Goyal to review progress and possibly end the BMT outpatient transplant process. Then at 60 days from transplant, I would return for bone marrow biopsy and more extensive blood testing to assess the state of cancer in my body and plan appropriate follow-up.

What about vaccinations? Laura said my flu shot could be obtained at 4 months after transplant, but all other immunizations (e.g., polio, Hepatitis B, measles, etc.) would wait until 6 months or later.

The central line removal was relatively uneventful. Dr. Martin removed a suture, applied local anesthetic, and simply pulled the line out of my chest. Irma watched the whole process! Although it sounded scary, it was quite painless. Dr. Martin assured us that I would not see serious bleeding because it does not look good for them if I leave a trail of blood on the floor.

When Irma and I got home, the garage was buzzing with ten Robo Raiders prototyping parts of their robot for this year's FTC robot game. They built models from cardboard, tape, and erector set pieces and powered them with motors and electric drills to see how they performed. After my encouraging BMT clinic visit, I interacted with the team and coaches without wearing a mask. It was good to be part of the action again.

Tuesday, September 11, 2018 (Transplant Day +25)

Tuesday began after generally good sleep with help from Tylenol PM. Irma and I were determined to do some work in the garden. Laura had okayed my doing work in the garden if I wore gloves and kept myself away from airborne contaminants that might carry fungi.

Irma and I worked for an hour hoeing and pulling weeds in an area by our back driveway. After a snack we went into my garden enclosure to clean up crop residue. Irma pulled out a corn row. I pruned back tomato plants and removed bad tomato fruit; then Irma and I picked good tomatoes. Irma pulled our green beans and harvested enough for our dinner. She also picked a few raspberries. I pulled our decimated cucumber plants. By 11 am we were both tired but also thankful for all that we had accomplished. Perhaps I was entering a period where I could do productive yard work again.

Irma and I took a nap after lunch. Robo Raiders came for their final 2 to 8 pm session of their robot-in-3-days challenge. I interacted with the team and other coaches without mask. At supper time Irma and I sat with the coaches as we enjoyed our food no longer in isolation.

September 12-16, 2018

Wednesday, September 12 followed a good night's sleep. I took no meds before bedtime and slept comfortably in our bed, not needing to go elsewhere to toss and turn. My body had its points of numbness and twinges of pain in some locations, but bothersome pain was not an issue.

Josh's brother Travis and his wife Margaret had to evacuate their North Carolina home to avoid Hurricane Florence, so they came to Mascoutah for a few days. Hearing Travis's (he is a nurse practitioner) stories about multiple myeloma, I was again thankful for my early diagnosis of MM and its rapid response to chemotherapy treatments.

Thursday began with a moderately good night's sleep. After a walk with Irma, I bought parts and repaired a toilet. Then Irma and I went shopping for groceries. I had a short nap after lunch. I continued preparation for my lesson on a quantitative method for analyzing game strategies, which I presented to the Robo Raiders later in the day. I helped Irma uncover the pool for swimming, then later covered it again. In all, this was a busy day and I had the energy to participate fully.

The remainder of the week I slept better, was active, and interacted with people without wearing a mask. I faithfully used hand sanitizer after shaking hands or touching things in public places. I was enjoying not having bangles dangling from my chest. I was not allowing my baldness to keep me from interacting with others.

On Friday, I received an email from Ron, director of the Iron Range Engineering program, expressing his sadness that I would no longer be involved in IRE. I told him that I had been experiencing the same sadness. Because I was now feeling very good and felt capable of traveling to the IRE meeting in just over a week, I indicated that I could attend if he desired.

This launched a flurry of discussions at home and with Ron to consider how best to proceed.

September 16 was my first day back at church without wearing a mask. I enjoyed visiting with people and recounting the amazing progress I had seen in answer to prayers of so many people. It was wonderful to sing without obstruction from a mask.

My first 30 days after the transplant had returned me to relatively normal health. During this time, I had experienced no medical emergencies that required me to make a sudden trip to the clinic or hospital. I had not even succumbed to common illnesses of people around me. I was feeling good about my recovery and hopeful that I would be doing all my normal things once again.

Partial Remission
Preparing for Maintenance

The Blood and Marrow Transplant clinic was looking to send me away after they had completed their transplant responsibilities. But before I would be discharged as an outpatient, they must determine that my blood composition had returned to normal and I was not showing signs of multiple myeloma. At 30 days and 60 days after the transplant, they wanted me to return to the clinic for tests and to review of my health status. When I became ready, they would send me back to Dr. Rodriguez for maintenance therapies until the next cancer flare-up occurred.

Monday, September 17, 2018 (Transplant Day +31)

September 17 was my 30-day checkup at the BMT clinic. After three tries, the nurses were able to draw blood samples so they could do basic multiple myeloma lab tests.

Results for this day (9/17) are shown compared to normal ranges and

COMPARISON OF 9/17/2018 to 7/2/2018 BLOOD COUNTS and LIGHT CHAIN PROTEINS			
Test	7/2/2018	9/17/2018	Normal
White cells	3.8	5.6	3.5-10.5
Red cells	4.33	**3.54 (L)**	4.30-5.70
Hemoglobin	**12.7 (L)**	**11.5 (L)**	13.5-17.5
Platelets	161	221	150-400
Neutrophil Absolute	3.3	2.6	1.6-7.0
Free Kappa Lt Chains	19.4	12.6	3.33-19.4
Free Lambda Lt Chains	10.0	6.3	5.7-26.3
Ratio Kappa/Lambda	**1.94 (H)**	**2.00 (H)**	.26-1.65

to values at the end of my June chemo treatments (7/2). My white cell count, platelets, neutrophil absolute, free kappa, and free lambda values were within normal ranges. Red cells and hemoglobin were low; the ratio of kappa to lambda light chains was a bit high. I was told that the high ratio was not of concern when occurring after the transplant.

An additional test, immunofixation serum, was conducted as another means of identifying the presence of cancer. Results shown indicated a normal pattern, which was the desired state, detecting no myeloma cells.

Laura, Kim, and Dr. Goyal were very pleased with how well my body had responded to the transplant process. We

> Serum immunofixation electrophoresis shows polyclonal IgG, IgA, and IgM immunoglobins. No monoclonal immunoglobins detected. Non-secretory myeloma (NSM) cannot be excluded on the basis of this result. Measurements of serum free kappa and lambda immunoglobin light chains can identify up to 70% of patients with NSM.

were reminded that earlier genetic testing showed 17p gene deletion. With this cancer suppression gene deleted, I would have a higher risk of recurrence of multiple myeloma.

I was told that during my next checkup on Transplant Day +60, more extensive testing would be done to assess the presence of multiple myeloma. The staff decided they would not do a bone marrow biopsy since they would have enough other test data. The likely return of multiple myeloma was at first frightening, but I reminded myself that God would be with me to direct what happens and would enable me to stand firm as I pass through any trials that arose.

After the 60-day checkup, I would probably be discharged by the clinic and be sent back to Dr. Rodriguez for maintenance therapies. Maintenance might include Revlimid at a lower dose than before and a bi-weekly injection of Velcade or related drug. I was glad to see that Dexamethasone was not included because in the past it kept me from sleeping.

Dr. Goyal also told us that two of her children were very interested in FIRST® robotics. This conversation followed from our earlier discussions of my robotics involvement.

After returning home I prepared for the Iron Range Engineering advisory board meeting. Ron and Christine wanted me to attend. I told Ron I felt that I had 90% of normal energy and was able to travel to the meeting by taking 2 days to drive each way. Reenergized by being a part of the IRE action, I set about to plan my travel.

September 18-21, 2018

On September 18 we started the Robo Raiders meeting with a team discussion of how to emulate their team Bible verse (1 Timothy 4:12):

> *"Don't let anyone look down on you because you are young, but set an example for the believers in speech, in conduct, in love, in faith and in purity."*

I was pleased to see how thoughtfully the students discussed the topic and identified how to be successful, then at the end of the 3-hour meeting reflected on their performance during work time. I had patterned this discussion after my college-level "mighty minutes" just-in-time professional development activities that were the core of my books. The team planned to continue discussions of professional and spiritual topics at meetings in the future so they would grow professionally as they engaged in robotics. I was pleased that my professional development contribution to the team was bearing good fruit.

September 20 I had a telephone meeting with Peter and Bashirah regarding our NSF grant at OSU. In this meeting I entered back into the work of the grant, which I had neglected for weeks.

Later that day, I researched multiple myeloma in patients who had 17p gene deletion. In such patients, multiple myeloma returned sooner and it more quickly became unresponsive to therapies. Life expectancy was reduced. This information made clear that my multiple myeloma was high-risk and the battle was not over. We must continue to trust God for the effectiveness of treatments and for strength to travel whatever path the Lord chooses for me.

Friday I participated in a video conference in an advisory capacity to a National Science Foundation project at New Mexico State University. During that call I was able to recognize a need and make a recommendation that the project leaders purposefully train students in skills they need to increase their success in engineering courses and stay in engineering programs. I again was encouraged to be able to contribute value to a research project.

September 23-26, 2018

On Saturday, September 23, Irma and I began a drive to Virginia, Minnesota for the Iron Range Engineering advisory board meeting. We drove 750 miles in two days and arrived for Sunday evening dinner with others on the advisory board. Driving that far was not hard on me.

All day Monday and Tuesday morning the advisory board met with students, faculty, and project facilitators to review the IRE program and identify recommendations for improving the program. I very much enjoyed working with the other advisors, learning about the program, and seeing solid capabilities of students in the program. To my surprise, I was recognized for my 10 years of service on the board, and a project room was named in my honor. The photo shows Irma and me standing by a plaque posted (down low) by the Denny Davis Design Project Room.

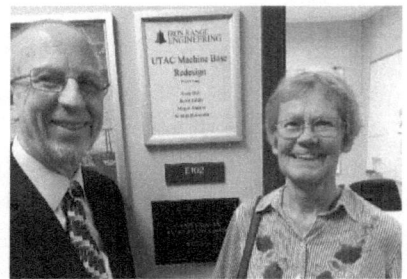

Irma and I traveled halfway home on Tuesday and the remainder on Wednesday. Again, driving long distances was not a problem.

Reflecting on my two advisory roles of the past week, I was greatly encouraged. My energy and ability to travel and make substantive contributions in engineering education was not noticeably affected by multiple myeloma.

September 27 – October 4, 2018

After returning from our Minnesota trip, Irma and I worked in the yard and garden to clean up plant debris and get the pool ready for winter. We found in the evening that Irma experienced pains in the shoulder, ribs, and back that probably resulted from overexertion doing yard work. Josh and his kids helped us cover the pool and blow water out of pipes for the winter.

After a successful Minnesota trip, we began reconsidering our earlier decision not to attend Irma's family's gathering near London, Ontario. Because I had traveled well and did not suffer from the long days in a car, I felt that I could similarly handle the 1000 miles of driving each way to the family gathering.

On September 30 (Sunday), Irma and I decided to make the trip to Ontario. I emailed Irma's family to inform them of our change in plans. We were trusting that God would keep both of us in good health for the trip and especially while in Canada.

Life seemed to have returned to normal. I was not having pain or struggling with sleep. My energy was nearly normal. But I used caution when working outside and when near sick people. Because I was presumably susceptible to sunburn, I wore my straw hat when in the sun for any period of time.

October 5-7, 2018

On Friday, after a walk and loading our car, Irma and I drove off to Lapeer, Michigan for the first day of our trip to Ontario. I drove through heavy rain and slow traffic at times but I was not overly exhausted by the driving.

Saturday morning I drove us to Alan and Margaret's farm near Ilderton, Ontario. We enjoyed visiting with relatives and delighting in my ability to travel to the event. I expressed my thankfulness that God had taken me through my multiple myeloma experience so painlessly. I stayed inside to avoid exposure to farm animals, but otherwise participated fully in family food and fun. We noted that my lack of hair was not much different from the hair sported by three of Irma's nephews.

After leaving the family gathering, I drove us to Flint, Michigan for night. Sunday morning I drove to Pullman, Michigan where we bought five 9-pound buckets of natural peanut butter to replenish our supply at home. Then we stopped for dinner in South Haven and drove home in time for supper. I was again pleased that I was able to travel without suffering from sickness or exhaustion. Thank you, Lord!

October 8-14, 2018

The next week was a mix of miscellaneous activities and waiting for my 60-day checkup. Irma and I hoed weeds in the yard and garden. We got our car serviced and made appointments for medical needs.

Robo Raiders continued to meet at our home in regular and extra work sessions as they prototyped their design ideas. Deadlines were approaching for them to select the best concepts and begin building their competition robot. On October 10, they invited two engineering professionals to our garage to review prototypes and give suggestions for their game strategy and design concepts. They received excellent input for guiding the team's robot design.

Knut had autumn break Thursday, October 11 through the weekend. Before leaving campus, he attended a career fair, where he hoped to find contacts for possible employment for the coming summer. Nancy drove to get him on Wednesday while Irma covered transportation needs for grandchildren going to music lessons.

This week some unusually warm weather ended, and cooler fall temperatures hit. With my bare head, I began wearing my new winter hat with ear flaps when I went for morning walks. Working in the garden also called for a warm hat. I suddenly realized that my sparse hair was leaving my head chilled even indoors. With this insight, I ordered a cap advertised for chemo patients to wear in daytime as well as at night. I had not really thought about needing head covering day and night, indoors and out. I had to prepare for my new image as "the short guy with a slouch beanie hat."

I continued working on my multiple myeloma story to get it into publishable form. Having earlier read Tom Brokaw's book, *A Lucky Life Interrupted*, I saw how a personal account could help prepare others to go through multiple myeloma. I wanted to add my book to those available to multiple myeloma patients, giving a different perspective on hope available during and after the cancer experience. With a nearly complete draft of my book in hand, I contacted Megan at SLUH to see if she continued to be interested in my book. To my delight, she was! I printed a draft to take to her during my Day +60 visit to SLUH. I hoped my book had value in the cancer treatment arena.

After nearly 60 days since my transplant, I was sleeping very well, not experiencing any pain or discomfort from the transplant. However, I began noticing discomfort when I lay on my left shoulder at night and it popped. This reminded me of physical therapy I had undergone a year earlier after injuring my shoulder while building fence. I recalled the therapist saying that I must keep my shoulder muscles in good condition to avoid similar injuries. This made me think seriously about regular strengthening exercises, which I had been avoiding. On October 13, I dug out rubber exercise bands I had used for therapy and began regular shoulder strengthening exercises.

Tuesday, October 16, 2018 (Transplant Day +60)

Tuesday, October 16 was 60 days after my stem cell transplant and a big day for checking my cancer status. Irma and I met with Laura at 11:30 am for blood draws and other tests to see if signs of multiple myeloma were returning. Mattie skillfully drew 5 vials of blood for tests after another nurse's attempt missed the vein.

After lunch Laura examined me and reviewed available test results with us. My blood chemistry was good. White cells and neutrophil absolute counts were within normal ranges. Red cells were a bit low but had increased from the previous month. Platelets had dropped just below normal. Laura said that overall counts looked good.

Laura questioned me about having any physical problems: pain, nausea, diarrhea, rash, appetite, sores, and swelling. I had none of these. I pointed out some small bumps on the back of my neck, which she examined and suggested we watch in the next few weeks. Thankfully, none of the common symptoms of myeloma were present.

I told Laura how pleased I had been with the care I received while an inpatient and as an outpatient. Based on my experiences, the BMT program provided excellent care.

Wednesday, October 17, 2018 (Transplant Day +61)

Wednesday morning I had an appointment for a long-overdue eye examination. In the exam I had difficulty reading both distant and nearby printed text, even with corrective lens adjustments. (My right eye had no useful vision because it was damaged in previous retinal detachment and reattachment.) After Dr. Walsh examined my eyes, he said that a cataract in my left eye was clouding my vision and preventing correction with refractive lenses. I needed the cataract removed before my vision in that eye could be improved.

I made an appointment for a pre-cataract surgery evaluation with Dr. Edelstein, who previously surgically removed a pterygium on my left eye. Even though cataract surgery was quite routine today, surgery on my only good eye was a bit concerning. I wondered what complications I might face with eye surgery and chemo possibly occurring in the same period of time. Clearly, we must trust God through this surgery.

In the afternoon, I found new BMT test results for blood cell counts and light chain protein analysis. As shown, the Lambda chains dropped significantly from the previous month and were well outside the normal range.

9/17/2018 to 10/16/2018 BLOOD COUNTS & LT CHAIN PROTEINS			
Test Result	**9/17/2018**	**10/16/2018**	**Normal**
White cells	5.6	5.9	3.5-10.5
Red cells	**3.54 (L)**	**4.01 (L)**	4.30-5.70
Hemoglobin	**11.5 (L)**	13.5	13.5-17.5
Platelets	221	**146 (L)**	150-400
Neutrophil Absolute	2.6	3.4	1.6-7.0
Free Kappa Lt Chains	12.6	9.8	3.33-19.4
Free Lambda Lt Chains	6.3	**2.8 (L)**	5.7-26.3
Ratio Kappa/Lambda	2.00 (H)	3.50 (H)	.26-1.65

The Kappa/Lambda ratio moved further above the normal range than in the previous month. Platelets had drop significantly this month. These changes caused me to wonder if they were indications of myeloma. To really understand these results, we would wait until our meeting with Dr. Goyal.

After returning home, my hat arrival caused my headwear to take on a new look for the cooler months. I began wearing a floppy beanie indoors to keep my bare head from chilling drafts while at my computer, napping, just moving through the house, or in bed at night. I did not want sinus infections or a cold. I found my beanies very comfortable and cozy, though they didn't make a stunning fashion statement. I had not expected that multiple myeloma might affect my wardrobe and my image in this way.

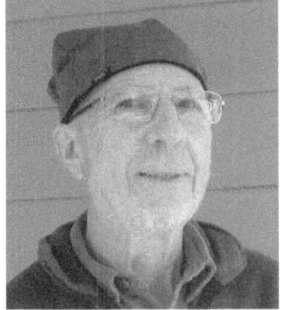

Saturday, October 20, 2018 (Transplant Day +64)

Saturday, October 20 was a big day for the small town of Mascoutah. Its annual Fall Fest blocked Main Street for displays, vendors, chili tasting, and a car show. Our Robo Raiders set up a display to represent FIRST® to the community, promote their team, and develop their abilities to communicate with the public. They showed robots from the previous year, a 3D printer in action, robot side plates cut with a CNC milling machine,

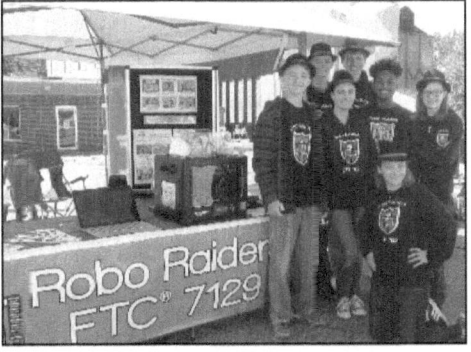

and displays of their outreach and robot design process. They did an outstanding job, even with a strong wind blowing things around. The photo shows seven members working the morning shift.

It was a lovely sunny day for mid-October. All 10 of our team members and 5 mentors/coaches represented the Robo Raiders at different times during the day. I enjoyed interacting with our team and people from the community without a mask. I limited my time in the sun to comply with a warning on my sulfamethoxazole pill bottle, another minor impact of multiple myeloma.

Sunday, October 21, 2018 (Transplant Day +65)

Sunday was busy with our early morning walk, church, a bike ride, reviewing family estate issues, and attending a missionary presentation. In church I sensed that people were more willing to interact with me, not staying away to keep from exposing me to germs. Many times I stated that I was feeling very normal and had full energy back. I received comments that I was looking better, with normal energy and good color. I think the sunshine helped to brighten my complexion.

Sunday evening I received feedback from Megan regarding the draft book I had lent to her. She was very encouraging. I was pleased that my medical descriptions were accurate and that Megan felt my book might be of interest to many staff working with cancer patients.

Monday, October 22, 2018 (Transplant Day +66)

On Monday, Irma and I met with Laura, Kim, and Dr. Goyal at the SLU BMT outpatient clinic. I had compiled blood test data so I could ask about platelets, red blood cell counts, and the Kappa/Lambda ratio that seemed to be outside normal ranges. Dr. Goyal quickly diffused my concerns about the test data by saying that all of my lab test results were wonderful. Their team was happy with my results.

Dr. Goyal explained that platelets vary a lot and should not be a concern. Red cells and hemoglobin were low but they had steadily increased, as was desired. The Kappa and Lambda light chain proteins were being interpreted by a new calculation based on their differences; this calculation looked good and should get better with time. There were no concerns!

I was being discharged from BMT with a status: VGPR, or very good partial remission. Partial was because some proteins had not had adequate time to reach their final state following the transplant. This should occur in the next few weeks.

I was being referred to Dr. Rodriguez for maintenance therapy. Therapy would likely be as suggested earlier: 10 mg/day of Revlimid, an injection of Velcade every 2 weeks, an infusion of Zometa for bone strength every 3 months. This regimen would continue until my body could not handle treatment toxicity or multiple myeloma failed to respond to treatments. At that point I would return to SLU BMT for additional testing and modification of the treatment plan.

When I asked about possible complications around cataract surgery, Laura assured me that I should not encounter complications due to concurrent chemotherapy treatments.

Later in the day I commented to Irma that I had worn to our meeting my jacket with a patch commemorating my climb of Mount Adams in June 1970. (See photo with me atop Mt Adams). I wondered if I was going to be fit enough for that kind of physical challenge in the future.

October 23-26, 2018

Tuesday I took steps to get my Verity Design Learning website operational. I transferred my domain name, VerityDesignLearning.com, to a wix.com server where I had created new content. I was overjoyed to get the new site operational and promote my books and other resources. I also placed a "coming soon" entry that refers to my multiple myeloma story.

The next day Dr. Rodriguez' office called with November 7 appointments for my maintenance therapy. That evening I sent an update on my health to family and friends via a number of email groups. The next day I got a call that set up delivery of Revlimid for a month of therapy.

Wednesday morning my throat started hurting, and it worsened throughout the day. I felt that a cold was on its way. If I had gotten a cold during my inpatient or early outpatient periods when white cell counts were low, I would have been vulnerable to serious complications. Since my white cell counts were normal this week, I was not overly concerned. However, I wondered how a cold might develop and persist when my immunities were probably nonexistent.

Thursday morning Irma and I were ready to drive to Branson for our rendezvous with my brothers and their wives. But when I woke, I had a cold and my voice was very deep. We ate breakfast anticipating a 7 am departure. As we discussed concerns about my health and impacts of a sick person on others, we decided to stay home. An hour later I had a change of mind, and we decided to start the drive to see how I traveled. We kept going and got to Branson in time for a late lunch with the others.

My cold was a bother during this trip, but it did not develop into a serious health concern. My highest temperature was 99.9F, not a dangerous level. Thursday afternoon and night the cold was mostly in my throat, and I was never badly congested. Friday I had a lot of sinus drainage but no restricted breathing.

We were able to spend very enjoyable times with family on Thursday afternoon and Friday morning. We drove home Friday afternoon, with Irma doing most of the driving. Once home, Irma got me some decongestant and I slept well. By Saturday, the drainage was greatly reduced and I was feeling reasonable. Irma and I went for a bike ride in the afternoon. We also had Josh and Nancy and their kids over for dinner, although I still had a noticeable cold. It appeared that my body was recovering well from this first illness after my transplant.

Reflecting on the past few days, Irma and I realized that we had become lax in our sanitation. In recent days we had had in our home Robo Raiders and family members with colds, and we had not sanitized thoroughly afterward. Yes, my body seemed to be able to handle sickness, but we should be more careful to prevent illness. The next illness might be much more serious. Thank you, Lord, for a gentle reminder to be careful.

End of October, 2018 (transition)

As October 2018 drew to an end, my multiple myeloma battle was transitioning from targeted intense treatments to general maintenance therapy. The battle began months earlier to stop a multiple myeloma attack on my skull. Chemotherapy and a stem cell transplant drove this cancer into remission, but it likely was not destroyed. It could be lurking in the shadows for another vicious attack. Having invaded bones in the past, it likely would attack bones in the future.

My high-risk 17p gene deletion left me vulnerable to future attacks and possibly new treatment challenges. We did not know when or where multiple myeloma might strike next, but we could expect that it would be back.

Up to this point, my multiple myeloma journey was supported by a talented medical team, dedicated family, and many people praying for me. Every step of the way, I was spared dreadful conditions commonly experienced by cancer patients. Mine had been an amazing hope-filled journey!

In order to face my uncertain future, we must confidently hold onto the hope that proved potent before. We had assurances that God was in control; He still is. He stood by us and enabled us to prevail in struggles; He will do so again. We know that God can destroy any attacker that might come against us, and yet God lovingly uses trials to prepare us for the future.

We clearly need this God of hope who brings us joy and peace as we trust in Him . . . for the short term and for all of eternity. Read on to learn how this hope is acquired.

A Sure Hope
Holding onto an Anchor

Living more than eight months with multiple myeloma gave me many trials for proving that my hope was sure. For each trial or fear faced, I found comforting assurances from the Bible, which were followed by events confirming these assurances. Examples are given below.

1. **Cancer discovery** [received shocking cancer diagnosis]
   <u>Assurance</u>: *Don't worry about anything; instead, pray*[1]
   <u>Outcome</u>: Treatable cancer found before bad bone/organ damage
2. **Cranial surgery** [faced risky, delicate procedure]
   <u>Assurance</u>: *The peace of God ... will guard your hearts and minds*[2]
   <u>Outcome:</u> Tumor removed without bad pain or loss of sensory, motor, or cognitive function
3. **Chemotherapy** [10+ week treatment with 3 kinds of chemo]
   <u>Assurance</u>: *The Lord goes before you ... Do not be afraid*[3]
   <u>Outcome:</u> Cancer rapidly went to remission; minimal side effects
4. **Transplant eligibility** [must make life-altering decision]
   <u>Assurance</u>: *Trust the Lord with all your heart, lean not on your own understanding*[4]
   <u>Outcome</u>: Testing decisively proved my eligibility for transplant
5. **Stem cell collection** [delicate collection; unknown duration]
   <u>Assurance</u>: *God of hope fill you with all joy and peace as you trust him*[5]
   <u>Outcome</u>: Stem cells extracted 2 days provided for two transplants

---

[1] Philippians 4:6
[2] Philippians 4:7
[3] Deuteronomy 31:8
[4] Proverbs 3:5-6
[5] Romans 15:13

6. **High-dose chemotherapy** [two days of very potent chemo]
   Assurance: *Though I walk through the darkest valley, I will fear no evil for You are with me*[6]
   Outcome: Chemo infused smoothly, no reactions or complications
7. **Stem cell transplant** [reintroduce stem cells that must engraft]
   Assurance: *In Christ, he is a new creature ... new things have come*[7]
   Outcome: Stem cells infused painlessly, engrafted in 10 days
8. **Neutropenia** [live under weakened, very susceptible condition]
   Assurance: *He gives power to the weak; to those who have no might He increases strength*[8].
   Outcome: Maintained energy; no infections or complications
9. **Outpatient care** [take new responsibilities; learn new limits]
   Assurance: *God comforts us so we can comfort others*[9]
   Outcome: Calmly managed pain and sleep, and travelled widely without serious problems or emergencies

My journey from cancer diagnosis to recovery after stem cell transplant showed me that short-term hopes are fulfilled even as we wait for our eternal hope. But we must understand the basis for our hope and take hold of hope that is more than luck or a positive attitude about the inevitable. Real hope is knowing that promises of good outcomes will be fulfilled.

Where is Real Hope Found?

Real hope stands on conditions that will unfailingly deliver good outcomes. We might gain hope from skillful medical professionals using proven practices. We might find hope in caregivers standing with us through hard times. Our own obedience to doctors' instructions and practicing good personal care add hope. But these sources of hope are unreliable: people have imperfect knowledge and inadequate will or ability to deliver.

---

[6] Psalm 23:4
[7] 2 Corinthians 5:17
[8] Isaiah 40:29
[9] 2 Corinthian 1:3-4

Unshakable hope requires someone with complete knowledge making wise decisions and executing perfect plans flawlessly. Only the God who created the universe and crafted us knows intricacies of our makeup, medical history, and how we respond to cancers and to treatments. He knows our needs better than we do. And He can deliver precisely what is needed to achieve good outcomes.

The God of the Bible is the source of my hope. My confidence is based on the reliability of the Bible, God's character as revealed in the Bible, and many examples of God's faithfulness in delivering good outcomes. I have had many hopes realized since I came to know and trust God in 1969. He is the God of hope who can give us peace and joy as we trust in Him.

What Hope is Available?

Facing cancer, we hope for painless treatments that quickly and permanently remove the dreaded disease from our bodies. We also hope for extended life, restored function and stamina, freedom from debilitating fears, and regrowth of hair. Some of us also hope for greater faith in God to face other threats.

Our hope begins by knowing that God loves us and plans what is truly best for us. God wants our lives to gain meaning as we personally know, enjoy, and worship Him. He desires that each of us would spend eternity with Him, free from pain and suffering and engulfed in happiness.

As stated at the start of my story, God uses trials to build our perseverance to prepare us better for the future. But even if He delivers us from suffering now, God will help us grow in our relationship with Him and live lives of hope. For our eternal good, we must join Him before we die.

Here are some hopes we have based on Bible promises:
- Shepherding—He protects and guides the weak
- Presence—He never leaves nor forsakes His children
- Enabling—He gives strength and wisdom if we ask
- Healing—He heals people, whom and how He chooses
- Knowledge—He reveals His nature, ways, desires for us
- Relationship—He is near us when we submit to Him

How Do I Access this Hope?

We access the hope offered by God when we stop playing God and let Him take charge in our lives. When God is in control, He can work our trials into hope-filled outcomes. First we must ask God (pray) that He will remake us and take control of our lives, as outlined below.

Acknowledge God as God. We acknowledge God as God when we agree that He rightfully has authority over the world and us. God is pure, right, loving, and expecting obedience. He defines what is true and what makes us acceptable to Him. We must relinquish any notion that we can tell God what is true or right. Instead, we must tell Him that we see Him as the only true God.

Admit our unworthiness. We recognize our unworthiness when we see ourselves accurately in contrast to God. All of us have disobeyed God, ignored Him, rejected His ways, or even defiantly fought Him. Our failures have separated us and erected an unscalable spiritual barrier between us and God. We cannot enter God's presence, and we do not deserve His work to remake us into what we really should be. In prayer we must admit to Him our many shortcomings and our failure to meet His perfect standards.

Accept God's currency. We must accept God's payment plan that requires a new kind of currency to pay for our transgressions. Our debt is far greater than we could pay. God declares that the only sufficient payment comes from Him: He sent His Son Jesus Christ, whose sacrificial death was sufficient to "pay-in-full" the debt of the whole world. We must agree with God that this sacrifice is the only acceptable currency for paying our spiritual debt to God.

Submit our life to Jesus. Finally, we must take action to complete a transaction with God. We must accept the offered payment for our debts, and yield ourselves to Jesus, God's Son. Then we are purchased by God and we no longer hold the reigns to our lives. We become a child of God, who has an inheritance in heaven. As one of His special people, God works all things to good ends for us, both now and eternally. We must verbalize to God our acceptance of His payment and our submission to Jesus Christ. We should also tell others about our decision.

For more information about getting to know God and Jesus Christ and about growing in our faith, see:

https://peacewithgod.net/ or

https://www.teenmissions.org/resources/abcs-salvation/ or

https://www.cru.org/us/en/how-to-know-god/would-you-like-to-know-god-personally.html

With a sure hope for today and for all of eternity, we can face troubles without being defeated! This requires that we get to know Jesus Christ intimately by reading about Him in the Bible and praying to Him. (If you are just getting started, read the book of Mark or the book of John in the Bible). We need to sit under sound Bible teaching and gather with others who share our present and eternal hope through Jesus Christ. With these anchors, we can encourage one another and bring glory to God as we collectively stand with Him in battles. We can victoriously battle multiple myeloma or any other challenges with the help of God.

www.ingramcontent.com/pod-product-compliance
Lightning Source LLC
Chambersburg PA
CBHW031432210526
45464CB00005B/2163